Angela's Decision

Also from Angela Schmidt Fishbaugh:
Seeking Balance in an Unbalanced World: A Teacher's Journey
Celebrate Nature! Activities for Every Season

www.balanceteacher.com

Angela's Decision

Outsmarting My Cancer Genes and Determining My Fate

Angela Schmidt Fishbaugh

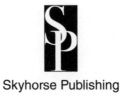

Skyhorse Publishing

Skyhorse Publishing books may be purchased in bulk at special discounts for sales promotion, corporate gifts, fund-raising, or educational purposes. Special editions can also be created to specifications. For details, contact the Special Sales Department, Skyhorse Publishing, 307 West 36th Street, 11th Floor, New York, NY 10018 or info@ skyhorsepublishing.com.

Skyhorse® and Skyhorse Publishing® are registered trademarks of Skyhorse Publishing, Inc.®, a Delaware corporation.

Visit our website at www.skyhorsepublishing.com.

10 9 8 7 6 5 4 3 2 1

Library of Congress Cataloging-in-Publication Data

Fishbaugh, Angela Schmidt.
  Angela's decision: outsmarting my cancer genes and determining my fate/Angela Schmidt Fishbaugh.
    pages cm
  ISBN 978-1-63220-473-8 (hardback)—ISBN 978-1-63220-740-1 (ebook) 1. Fishbaugh, Angela Schmidt—Health. 2. Breast—Cancer—Genetic aspects. 3. Ovaries—Cancer—Genetic aspects. 4. Breast—Cancer—Prevention. 5. Ovaries—Cancer—Prevention. 6. Breast—Cancer—Patients—United States—Biography. 7. Ovaries—Cancer—Patients—United States—Biography. 8. BRCA genes. I. Title.
  RC280.B8F563 2015
  616.99'449042—dc23
                           2014039509
Cover design by David Sankey

Print ISBN: 978-1-63220-473-8
Ebook ISBN: 978-1-63220-740-1

Printed in the United States of America

Dedication

This book is dedicated to you, the reader.
I have felt your loss and now your joy. Together we heal!

With love to all my family and friends!

Note to the Reader:
I have changed many of the names in this book, including all of
the health care workers—those professionals that offered me their
opinions, performed medical tests, and the doctors that did my
surgeries. These names have been changed for obvious reasons.

I have also changed the names of some of the people who
came into my life for a short time and were, for the most part, my
tolerance testers. All tolerance testers have made me a stronger
person and, as you will discover, my inner dialogue speaks frankly
about these issues. But truthfulness sometimes doesn't paint the
prettiest picture, so these names have been changed as well.

I hope you always speak your truth!

Contents

Introduction   ix

Preface: The Pensive Hours before Surgery   xiii

1. Mind, Body, Spirit, and Preschool Mealtime   1
2. Roots of Compassion   9
3. "Thank God This is Only an Office Procedure"   21
4. The Twists and Turns of Waiting   31
5. Testing for My Legacy   37
6. In My Own Shoes   53
7. "Inspired"   79
8. Surgery and Pain (Meds)   91
9. V for Victory, V for Visitors   111
10. Bereavement and Resolutions   131
11. Changing, Inside and Out   139
12. Caring for the Girls   151
13. The Lows of the High   157
14. The New Woman   163

Epilogue   179

Resources   181

Acknowledgments   183

Introduction

I am positive for *BRCA1*, a gene that gives me over an eighty percent chance of getting breast cancer and over a forty percent chance of getting ovarian cancer in my lifetime. I am now what is called a "previvor,"[1] which means I've never had cancer; however, I still have the genetic traits which increase my chances of getting cancer. I am a previvor because I opted to have two preventative operations, and as is the case with any major operation, there were ramifications. But, thanks to my decision to have these operations, I now have reduced my chances of ever getting cancer by ninety percent. This book takes you on that journey—from deciding to get genetically tested (because five of my closest relatives died of cancer at a very young age) to the decisions made during that difficult period of my life.

I originally wanted to write this book to help women understand genetic testing and proactive surgeries. Now that the book is finished, I realize that it does so much more than that. It is here to take you on a journey; not just my journey, but one that is yours as well. Anyone who has ever witnessed a loved one fight cancer knows all too well about that powerful journey you go through together. Although each journey is unique and poignant, our stories intertwine with parallels of courage, quiet tears, and touching moments.

The journey is also about growing as a person. Within these pages, you will uncover deep feelings of loss—whether it is the loss of a loved one or the ability to do what you were once able to do—and joy, like that of being a mother, a daughter, and the best person you can be while alive on this earth. It is through the discovery of these feelings that we are able to move more freely in life.

So this book is for you. Here's to our journey together. I am certain you will cry and laugh and sing and hopefully paddle (you'll understand what this means later), and more importantly, I hope you always make the decision to live your best life!

Blessings and Love,
Angela

---

1. The term "previvor" was coined in 2000 by Facing Our Risk of Cancer Empowered. Previvors are those individuals who have a predisposition to cancer and take action to reduce the possibility of its occurrence. More information can be found in the resources section.

A Moment inside My Journey

by Angela Schmidt Fishbaugh
December 30, 2009

Phone ringing
Need testing
More investigating
Gripping, holding, waiting

Results shocking
Anger crying
No reassuring
Questioning, denying, weeping

Facts researching
Life missing
Graciously deciding
Recognizing, preventing, accepting

Information sharing
People loving
Procedures approaching
Trusting, hoping, fearing

Through awakening
Painful hurting
Emotional wounding
Suffering, feeling, sensing

Thoughtfulness pouring
Kindheartedness filling
Gifts overwhelming
Sighing, receiving, healing

Again Preparing
Reject wondering
Appreciate knowing
Understanding, valuing, loving
a moment inside my journey

Preface

The Pensive Hours before Surgery

December 3, 2009

Lying in my tub, I try to keep my upper body from being submerged in the water. By my doctor's orders, my breasts are not allowed under the water. There are purple circles around each nipple that stretch length-wise and outward, making my small breasts look like someone has drawn large, purple eyes on them. Water-resistant skin tape covers them, creating an unsightly wrinkled look. I look at my taped breasts and begin to cry. It's 4:00 a.m., and my breasts will be removed this morning.

"I won't be attached to you. I need to be attached to life," I say to myself. I have made the decision to have a bilateral mastectomy, and I will have a total hysterectomy eight weeks from now. I have made this decision not because I have cancer but because I have tested positive for a rare cancer gene, called *BRCA1*. All four doctors within a hundred-mile radius of my home, from whom I have recently received opinions, have given me the same heartrending diagnosis, and each affirms that the longer I wait to do anything about it, the more likely it will be that cancer comes knocking on my door.

The nickname in the medical community for my Hereditary Breast and Ovarian Cancer syndrome (HBOC) is "Early Onset," and because I am forty-one years old, "early onset" is yesterday or a few minutes from now. The most alarming statistic is that my precious, innocent children—my beautiful and lively eight-year-old daughter and handsome and vibrant eighteen-year-old son—have a fifty percent chance of carrying the mutated gene as well. I have made the decision not to think about this latter fact, and I have made the decision to be attached to life.

It is quiet in my home. I press a warm washcloth against my face and breathe in the steam, being careful not to splash any water near my breasts. I hear my husband shuffling around downstairs as he makes coffee for our two hour trip to the hospital. Our daughter has stayed the night with a dear and longtime friend of mine so her school life can be as "normal" as possible, while our eighteen-year-old son rests in his bedroom. We will count on him to take care of our pets and home for the next few days. Since many of my own family members have died of cancer, I must rely on friends and immediate family for all the help I need during this time.

Getting out of the warm tub, I carefully dab the few droplets of water from my taped breasts. I stand naked, looking in the full length mirror at my thin build, and murmur my mantra: "A mediocre decision made in a timely manner is better than a perfect decision made too late." As I get dressed and put on my expensive 36B push up bra, tugging, tightening, and fixing it so the protective shell fits snuggly against my body, my thoughts run back and forth over whether I should wear this bra or go braless. *Maybe I should go braless. I could be sexy one last time.* I make the decision to wear the bra and wonder if sexy is a matter of the mind. I cling to this latter positive thought.

As I walk downstairs with my overnight bag this early December morning, I turn to my husband. "Okay, I think I'm ready," I say in as positive a manner as I can. Richard takes my bag and gently nods for me to say good-bye to Matt. I softly knock on his bedroom door and then walk in peacefully. "Matt, we're going, honey. Take care of the home." I'm proud to hear his reply. "I love you, Mom, let me give you a hug." As he stumbles out of bed to hug me tightly, I know that not only have I made the best decision, but I've also raised really good children. I decide, yet again, that I yearn to be around for my children's lives. This is the feeling I embrace as I hold my son close.

"I love you," I say to him.

"I love you too," he responds lovingly.

In the car, and as Richard backs out of the dark driveway, I set the GPS for the hospital and drink my coffee. I typically drink my coffee with wonderful flavors of frothy and heavenly cream, with names that include things like "mudslide" and "toffee." But today it's black, hard-hitting, and tough to take, just like the day that is unfolding before me. I was instructed to only have water, plain tea, or black coffee after midnight in preparation for today's operation. It was then that I took my last bite of lasagna and finished off yet another glass of red wine. I feel sorry for myself and complain about this fast to Richard. "The hospital food has gotten better, I've heard," he says, trying to reassure me. I drink more black coffee. Two hours to go. Two hours until the hospital exit.

I close my eyes and remember the day I went with my mother for her doctor's report appointment. I can see the doctor, now nearly ten years ago, as she told my mother her biopsy *did* reveal cancer tissue. Her doctor, a short, dark-haired woman who went to the same Episcopal Church that we sometimes went to, had come into our tiny examining room with her clipboard. I knew the diagnosis before she muttered a word; it was in her eyes, in the way she looked down to avoid our own anxious gazes. She came into the room and gave a brief nanosecond of a look towards us and a longer, deeper look at the infirmary's tile floor. Then she returned her gaze to my mother.

"Marlene," she said, "you have breast cancer. It has spread to your lymph nodes, but it is very, very small." The doctor emphasized this by holding up her hand and making a small space between her forefinger and thumb, trying to peek through it with her left eye. I sighed as the doctor strained to see through the miniscule opening between her tiny fingers and then straightened my spine in preparation for the emotional load ahead. The hospital surgeries, the follow-up appointments, and the exhausting daily phone calls from my mother would consume my home and work life for the next six months.

I open my eyes and sip some more of my now-lukewarm black coffee. I can feel coffee grounds in-between my teeth, which makes me want to spit. I realize I am angry and think that I shouldn't have to deal with this crappy and tepid black coffee. My anger moves to why someone like me has such a high chance of getting breast cancer. I mean, really? I am a pre-K teacher and a public service employee. I devote my life to teaching little ones to grow up and become strong citizens. Isn't that noble enough to be able to live a long life? I should be getting some kind of teacher award. Instead, I'm getting my breasts cut off. I calm myself by breathing and remind myself that the decision to have a mastectomy was my own. I think of the family that I need to take care of, and that love strengthens me. I wriggle the coffee grounds around in my mouth and long for all the little things that sweeten up life, like my hazelnut creamer and the boys and girls who hug me at school each day and say "I love you, Mrs. Fishbaugh."

"I believe we're the next exit," I say to Richard as I wipe a tear from my eye. The sounds of the wet highway and the dreariness of this cold winter day weigh heavily on me. I rest my head against the cold, foggy window and listen to the watery hissing of the highway as we pass over it. There is a solemn feeling in my heart.

This feeling isn't new to me and I have been taking trips to the hospital virtually my whole life. They really started when I had just turned nineteen years old, after my dad was first diagnosed with lung and brain cancer, and would continue as I helped my family deal with his, and later my mother's, fight against cancer.

I close my eyes and this time dredge up the memory of driving my mom to see a plastic surgeon. He had an office forty-five minutes from my mother's small town hospital where she had been diagnosed, and he was going to remove and reconstruct her right breast. When we arrived at his building, I had been completely surprised by the upper-crust feel of the structure. The lawn looked like artificial grass and the massive sculptures arranged on it were beautiful, abstract golden pieces. Before crossing the threshold of the entryway, my mother tossed her cigarette on the sidewalk and stepped on it. I rolled my eyes and pointed smugly at an ornamental cement ashtray next to the door.

"Oh, that's what that is for." She laughed and coughed uncontrollably and smiled the demented smile she wore when she was deliberately pissing me off. I rolled my eyes again, but this time with a grin.

We walked through the door and onto an emerald carpet. There were sumptuous paintings of women's figures in the lobby, and I remember thinking it could have been an art gallery instead of a doctor's office. This establishment's ambiance was the opposite of the hospital we had just come from; Mom had dressed for that setting, not this fancy one. She had on her blue jeans and long fleece button-up sweatshirt. Her oversized purse, which carried her numerous prescription bottles and extra packs of cigarettes, appeared heavier than usual.

A beautiful woman with long dark hair greeted us as she slid open the glass window of her little office.

"May I help you?"

"I have an—" my mother coughed and then composed herself enough to say "—appointment."

The woman's lip gloss looked freshly applied. "Your name?" she asked as she looked through her appointment book.

"Marlene," my mom coughed. "Marlene Schmidt."

My husband hits a pothole and I bounce upright, the jolt bringing me back into the present. It is still dark and I can feel my heart pounding so I close my eyes again. *My God, this day is really here*, I think to myself. Just yesterday afternoon, my best friends were sitting in my brightly colored pre-K classroom believing they were consoling me, when really I felt like I was consoling them. I tighten my eyes even more and reach for Richard's right hand as he takes the exit off the thruway. I can see my friends' faces; a bit scared but trying to appear confident. I smile and picture my friend Heywood conjuring up his most inappropriate jokes. The combination of his attempts at relieving the tension, my best friends' smiles, and the I love yous were just what I needed to prepare me for this all-too-serious event.

1

Mind, Body, Spirit, and Preschool Mealtime

August 18, 2009

I have my routine pap smear today. The one unusual feature is that I have chosen a midwife for the procedure, rather than a gynecologist. I like my midwife Beth very much; she's always seemed more alternative and radical than I am. She worked within a traditional hospital setting before venturing out on her own. I used to visit Beth when she was affiliated with the local hospital near my home, but now I travel ten or so miles to her new women's center. I've always thought it sounded better to say "I'm visiting my midwife for my annual well-woman-care appointment" versus saying "I'm visiting my gynecologist for my annual pap smear."

Beth's new center appears more spa-like than medical, which is a relief to me since I dislike feeling like a patient. Her spacious examining room has beautiful rock walls, serene music, and a chaise leather sofa with golden upholstery tacks. The resort atmosphere makes me feel comfortable as I climb onto the pelvic examining table. Soft leg warmers cover the metal stirrups where I rest my feet, and I cover myself with a blanket as Beth turns on the arm lamp and shifts it to better see between my legs. Despite my prone position, we continue our healthy therapeutic talk about our nourishing vegetable gardens and the benefits of red wine and wholesome natural supplements, all of which have connected us for years.

"So what else is new, Angela? Are you still doing lots of yoga? Would you consider teaching prenatal yoga here? I've just renovated the upstairs and we've already started HypnoBirthing classes."

Beth has been asking me to do prenatal yoga classes for the past few years and I always feel bad turning her down. Although I am a certified sports yoga instructor, I can't seem to muster up the carefree, be-in-the-moment yoga attitude required when working with pregnant women.

"Pregnant women and yoga scare me," I say to her.

Beth laughs. "You did yoga when you were pregnant."

"I know, but I didn't have to be responsible for anyone hurting themselves."

"I understand," she assures me, now beginning to give me her play-by-play down there. "Okay, Angela, take a deep breath and keep breathing. I'm just inserting the speculum." Then she taps it and adds "Okay, just a quick swab here." Beth then turns to her small metal prep table and fidgets with the swab and the glass slide.

I'm totally uncomfortable and grumble. "Are we done?"

"Almost, almost," she reassures. "And now one more swab from the cervix."

I'm holding my breath and all tensed up as usual during this part of the procedure.

"Now are we done?"

"Almost," Beth laughs, adding that I should relax and breathe.

I realize I'm all tightened up and take a deep breath. Then I literally feel the cervix swab, which is always the worst. She taps the metal speculum again and slowly takes it out. She then does her finger exam and uses her other hand on top of my pubic bone and pushes around here and there. She then turns off the bright lamp.

"We're all finished."

"Thank God!" I kid with her, my eyes still closed. "For the love of God, what we women have to go through on this earth!" I then ask if she would mind checking my breasts as well.

Beth had found a small cyst several years ago and, knowing my well-hidden anxiety about getting cancer, had sent me to a doctor in Rochester, New York. That doctor had assured me that it was only a cyst and that it would *never* turn into cancer, something I always liked to hear a doctor say, especially considering my family history.

I've always admired Beth's ambition and her idealistic vision of vibrant health and high self-esteem for women of all races, sizes, and ages. We share similar health stances: if your mind and spirit are healthy and if you feed your body wholesome foods that include lots of greens and a rainbow of colors, you will live a long, long time and not get cancer. Her new clinic reflects this mindset.

Beth examines my breast. "Okay, dear, you're good to go. Go ahead and get dressed."

"Thank you, Beth. Could you write me a prescription for some pain meds?" I'm a bit ashamed to ask for the Naproxen prescription for my imminent painful periods. Beth has always been into meditation, lavender oils, and chamomile teas to keep menstrual cramps at bay. I have been too but I have come to need about three Naproxen a month as well. I figure that, in the big scheme of things, three little Naproxen pills a month can't hurt anyone.

"Of course, Angela." She writes me the prescription. "We'll see each other next summer."

On the way home I stop at a store to buy a bottle of Cabernet Franc to celebrate another successful annual woman's visit. I've loved wine since I started drinking it, which was shortly after I got my first teaching job and after I gave birth to my daughter, Adele. It was around that particular time that I gave up drinking soft drinks at dinner time and went to drinking wine instead. Holding a wine glass made me feel sophisticated, and I'd swirl the red wine and smell its aroma.

Sophistication is something I've yearned for ever since I began raising children, a job I've truly never stopped doing. I was four when my brother was born and five years old when my sister came. Mom put me in charge of everything the adults were supposed to do; she had two jobs to work and then beer to drink in the evening. I didn't do a very good job of raising my younger brother and sister, but, hey, I was only five, so I cut myself some slack. My younger brother, who is in his late thirties, has never even had a sip of wine or any type of alcohol. My younger sister went to the other extreme and has had a problem with alcohol since she was fifteen years old. She has been in and out of rehab most of her life. Their lives include mostly self-inflicted suffering, which saddens me.

These thoughts are far from my mind right now, though. It's summer, giving me more reason to have a glass of wine and celebrate. I love my summer life, and one of my favorite activities is to sit on my patio that overlooks our fifteen acres of land and eat good food, drink good wine, and talk good talk. Ten months out of the year I eat my breakfast and lunch in my pre-K classroom full of three- and four-year-olds. It is the most undignified and unpleasant part of my job, yet one of the most important parts as well. Nothing ever slips by my proper-eating etiquette. I try to pack wholesome foods the night before while picturing a wonderful lunch in my classroom. However, mealtime mostly becomes an endless teaching time where I am eating with a lot of youngsters starving for manners. It also includes a great deal of educating with my mouth full. It seems as though I can't get by one school lunch without hearing bathroom words.

"Owen just farted," shouts Jenna, one of my few well-mannered students.

"Owen, just say excuse me," I say, after swallowing a bite of my couscous.

"Mrs. Fishbaugh, Jared just said poop," hollers Caitlin, who tattles all the time.

"Jared, please don't use bathroom words at the lunch table," I say, trying to get in another bite in as graceful a manner as possible. "Caitlin, just show him how to have good manners," I add, now with my mouth full.

"Mrs. Fishbaugh, Owen is showing me the food in his mouth," Jenna screeches.

I talk again with my mouth partway full, trying to chew my bite of couscous.

"Boys and girls, let's all practice closing our mouths while we eat."

I take another bite of my lunch and point to my closed lips, realizing I've just killed two birds with one stone: I get to have a peaceful bite of lunch and teach at the same time. A few of the children are trying this newfound skill when I hear a child pass gas next to me, and of course, the whole class bursts out in laughter.

"Okay, boys and girls, our bodies do that sometimes. All you need to do is just say excuse me."

Usually this is about the time my friend Heywood, the science teacher, enters my pre-K classroom. I love him because he actually wants to visit my room during lunch.

"Hi, Mr. Heywood, look what we're learning. Boys and girls, show Mr. Heywood how you can chew like big boys and girls."

There is a nanosecond of quiet as most of the children look up at him, chewing with closed mouths.

"Wow, you guys are so smart," he encourages. I stand up and as we walk away from the children, he whispers to me, "I don't know how you do this all day, Fishbaugh!" We quietly talk about some union business and then he says bye to my class. Just as he exits, I call him back and run to the doorway.

"Oh, Mr. Heywood?" I say. He meets me in the doorway and, with my back turned to the children, I stick out my tongue to show him the chewed-up spinach and couscous in my mouth.

"Oh, nice!" he smirks, trying to sound disgusted.

This is our humor, and it gets me through these days of non-stop teaching. I turn back to the children. "Okay boys and girls, let's finish up."

I've been teaching almost my whole life. Even at the age of four, I would prop my baby sister and brother up against the couch and play school with them. Into my adult career, everyone has told me how good I am at teaching, regularly telling me I'm a natural. There are things I love about teaching and there are things that are extremely difficult. I've always loved watching positive changes occur in those students who attempt new things and take risks with their learning. For instance, there are always little ones who are afraid to speak in a group when they start school in September, but by the end of the year, they will be using a microphone and singing songs in front of their peers. These are the moments when I think, *I can teach for twenty more years.*

For the most part, I have been lucky to experience the daily hugs from my students and to hear them say "I love you, Mrs. Fishbaugh." All of this outweighs the negative stuff. I sometimes wish that those head honchos who create all of the scripted curriculums and the overwhelming paperwork and assessments, and anyone who has tried to tell me how to do my job, could eat one meal with my students in the classroom. Not just for a short moment, but one full mealtime. I would even love to see them in my classroom for a full day, sitting on the carpet trying to teach an academic lesson to eighteen preschoolers who are still learning not to pick their noses in public.

I have worked on letting go of any anger in this area as I believe anger can manifest itself in the body as disease. It is an ongoing letting go and I continually thank God for the yoga that helps me cope with it. I let go, take deep breaths, and stretch, relaxing into the trust I have in my gut. This is what carries me through the daily grind of teaching. It also helps me to be spontaneous. All of this encompasses my program to stay balanced and healthy in today's teaching world.

Deep in my heart I have figured out why sitting outside on my patio on a summer evening eating grilled salmon and veggies with a good bottle of local Cabernet Franc feels like one of the best adult things to do in my world. I love being able to take a small bite of fish, close my eyes and feel its soft texture on my tongue, and then open my eyes, hear the birds chirping, and smell the aroma of my wine as I sip it. I am in the moment with everything; the sounds and the tastes. I am dignified, mindful, and in the moment.

Dignified is what I have been looking for most of my life. When I was young—about my students' age—my parents would also sit outside to eat. We kids had to be well-mannered while the adults made many ill-mannered slips. It was a little different from my current Cabernet Franc routine.

In 1974, my mom would be drinking Old Milwaukee with my uncle John, who had just returned home from Vietnam and was living with us. My dad would be in his white T-shirt, simultaneously smoking a cigarette and throwing a Frisbee to the four of us kids. My dad, looking very cool in his Elvis hairdo, would throw the Frisbee and have it skip off the cement with a slight bounce and back up to us. He could also catch the Frisbee behind his back, and do so with a cigarette in his mouth.

My uncle John usually let out a good burp over the grill as he'd announce "Dinner's ready" with a slur. Buttered steak, baked potatoes with sour cream, and iceberg lettuce would then be served on the kitchen table, all the lit cigarettes in ashtrays to the side. Yes, the surgeon general had determined ten years earlier that smoking was bad for your health, but you could still smoke on most airplanes until the mid-eighties; having cigarettes at the dinner table in the early seventies, our family was right in tune with most of America. We'd all then take our plates to the back porch and set them on our laps, my uncle nudging me and quietly offering the gristle from his plate so I wouldn't have to argue with my brother for it. He'd wink as he guzzled the last froth from his beer.

Our typical Sunday meals after Catholic Mass were a bit more dignified than our Saturday cookouts. Grandpa would recite his five minute prayer in Polish because he didn't speak any English. During the prayer, my older brother would try to make me squeal and get us into trouble by purposefully squeezing my hand underneath the table. I usually opted out of getting us into trouble and took the squeeze, because getting caught meant double trouble for me, the punishment being holding hands with my brother in the corner and doing the dishes as well.

So I would suffer through my family's Catholic prayer and looked forward to our casual cookout dinner on the back porch the following weekend. Sometimes my parents invited their friend Bob, who wasn't exactly known for his fine manners and would do things like leaning to one side and farting. "Take that to the bank," he'd say. The entire family would laugh, and though I'd be embarrassed, I'd laugh anyhow at its absurdity. Somehow, all this mealtime manner karma has followed me into my career.

Therefore, if I can have any form of dignity while eating, I like to do it with a glass of Cabernet Franc in my hand. I have even mastered the art of holding my beautiful wine goblet. I am determined to maintain poise at any mealtime I am a part of.

"Beth's business is beautiful. I love her passion for helping women," I say to my husband, holding my pinky out to one side as I sip some wine.

"How did it go today?" Richard asks.

"Oh, fine! Beth said I looked good and that she'll see me next summer."

"That's great," Richard adds as he finishes off the last of the salmon from his plate.

I look down at my plate and notice I am only halfway through. My son is finished and Richard is on seconds and I find myself slightly annoyed by their improper manners. Adele, now nearly eight years old, has done a pretty good job on her rice, broccoli, and fish. I think she likes this meal because the different foods don't touch, like the food in a casserole or lasagna might. She asks to be excused and runs to the swing set.

"Why do women have to have pap smears?" Matthew, my nearly grown high school senior, suddenly asks. I offer my quickest explanation of being proactive and on top of one's health. Uninterested, he stacks some dishes and takes them in the house.

Richard laughs. "You know how to clear the table! Talk about pap smears and we get to be alone."

"It's just so nice to have that behind me and the rest of the summer to relax," I say as I sip a bit more wine.

2

Roots of Compassion

October 1, 2009

It's burger night in the Fishbaugh home. I try to make the best of our super quick meal—it has to be quick because Adele's elementary school is having an open house this evening. Her school is the same school I graduated from back in 1986. It is also the same school my dad graduated from in 1965. Adele has trouble understanding why I teach at a school that is about twenty miles from our home. I've always explained that if I were to teach in my hometown district where my children attend school, I would have to be on guard about what I say and the opinions I share, mainly because I'd be an employee there as well as a parent. Every time I give this same explanation, though, I realize I've never really censored any of my opinions or thoughts anyway. I think the real reason is that I have just not wanted the people at my work to know every move my kids are making in school.

My children are wonderful but they have been challenging too. My son, Matt, has spent a lot of his senior year making sure his grade point average remains two-tenths under the GPAs of the top two students in his graduating class. This way, he won't have to give a speech as valedictorian or salutatorian. Then there's my daughter, Adele. She has gone through reams of paper in every math and language class but not because she has been taking notes on how to do math problems or how to edit her elementary essays. Rather, it's because Adele draws animated cartoon figures or comic strips during every waking moment at school. Well, at least every moment that the teachers aren't noticing her lack of attention.

"Matt, can you set the table?" I shout over the guitar amp blaring from his room. Matt has put a great deal of his energy into becoming quite the heavy-metal guitar player. I seriously can never tell if he is playing a Metallica CD on his stereo or if he himself is playing his guitar. He's developed into a teenage intellectual who plays heavy-metal Metallica music during most of his free time. He can also tell you virtually every piece of trivial knowledge about Metallica's lead singer, James Hetfield. In fact, I've been told so much information about Metallica that I have become a trivia buff of the heavy-metal band too. I know, for instance, that Hetfield was only sixteen years old when his mom died from cancer and that his "Mama Said" song came from that family suffering.

I knock again on Matt's door and shout even louder over the guitar amp. "Matt, I need you to set the table. Like now."

Adele runs through the kitchen and our dog Odie—who doesn't like commotion—barks and chases her around the kitchen island.

"Adele, go back upstairs and get your school clothes back on. You're not wearing those dirty play clothes to open house!"

With Adele still running in circles, I whirl around and yell to my husband. "Richard, can you pour drinks?" I'm so busy that I forget to say please or thank you.

Richard walks calmly into the kitchen. "You know that we don't have to be at the school at *exactly* six p.m. Open house is from six to seven thirty."

"Yeah, but if we get there early we can visit the book fair before the whole Dundee community fills the small room and we can hardly breathe."

Richard and I are best friends but we can also bicker with the best of them.

"Okay," I yell, "time to eat!"

The four of us hold hands as we sit around the table. The burgers are already on our plates and the warm french fries are on the stoneware in the center of the table. I take a deep breath to slow down.

"Let's say our family prayer," I say.

Somehow, the family's monotonous drone calms me. "Bless this food to our use, guide us and direct us in all your ways, Amen!" It is the prayer that Richard and I have decided to use as our typical family prayer. Of course we vary the prayer from time to time given any situations that need praying for, such as a relative's sickness or a friend's suffering. But this one in particular has become our what-to-say-when-we-are-in-a-hurry-and-have-to-gobble-up-our-dinner prayer.

I grew up Catholic and Richard took refuge in Buddhism when he was in his thirties. When we first met, I attended some of his Buddhist ceremonies and actually felt quite at home with them, as the rituals were quite similar to those of my Catholic upbringing. The Buddhist ceremonies had bread and wine for communion, just as in my Catholic church. However, in the Buddhist formal service, we would sit on zafu cushions and the bread was real bread, not like the blessed Catholic wafers that tasted like cardboard. Also, in the Buddhist service, the wine was served by pouring it into the palm of your hand. You slurped it from your hand, or if you didn't drink wine, like Richard, you'd swipe the wine over top of your head.

On this evening, I pour a glass of wine for myself and set it at the dinner table, something that is a routine practice. The wine is meant to be for later, a nightcap of sorts, but I take a few sips. I do it without thought and when I realize what I'm doing, I think, *Oooops! I'm going to my daughter's elementary open house this evening!* But I shrug off my feeling of guilt and take one more sip anyway. I leave the rest for a later nightcap.

It's hard to believe that our dinner is as pleasant as it is. I thought the rush of it all would make me angry and that I'd somehow slip into my usual once a week mealtime rant about how I need to have a peaceful meal and how that's all I really want in this world—a nice, dignified meal with a caring husband and respectful children. But there isn't time enough to get into that miserable space because before I know it, everyone is putting the ketchup and leftover fries away and Richard has started the dishes.

As we scramble to make the kitchen look tidy and as the kids get their coats on, the phone rings.

"I'll get it," I yell. "Adele, you get buckled in."

I look at the caller ID and see that it's Beth's private phone number. In the short one-thousand-millionth of a second that it takes me to press "talk," I feel my heart pound and my body heat up. I answer the phone with a nervous "Hello?"

"Hi, Angela, it's Beth," she says. I realize she's trying to sound normal. As I walk into my art room, I picture her on the other end of the line looking down at the floor tiles.

"What's going on, Beth?" I ask quietly as I unzip my coat.

"I received your pap results and they were abnormal. I know how on top of things you like to be so I sent the samples back to the lab for more information and it did show a high risk HPV issue. It's not one of the worst numbers, like HPV 16 or 18, but it is a rare one, HPV 53."

I sit down in my chair and feel my husband put his hand on my right shoulder.

"So what does this mean, Beth?"

"I'm going to send you to Dr. Dayes. He's really good with these issues. I'll request that he do a cervical biopsy as well as an endometrial biopsy."

"How quickly can I do all of this?" I ask without hesitation.

"Don't worry, we can get you scheduled quickly," Beth assures me.

"Okay then. Thanks for your call, Beth." I hang up the phone numbly.

"What's going on?" Richard asks. His tone is caring and loving. As I tell him about the phone call, I realize that Beth has referred me back to the same hospital that she walked away from several years before, the one that felt more like a hospital than a spa. I have always felt a little special for going to her new women's center. I had thought that by doing yoga and staying fit and healthy I could be a *client* in a contemporary women's center. I sense the medical feel of being a patient as I am referred back to the hospital. It leaves me feeling shaken.

"Come on, let's go to Adele's open house!" I say. As I leave my art room, I look up at the two banners above the doorway. The one in the center reads: DARE TO TAKE RISKS. The other smaller one to the right reads: SMOOTH SEAS DON'T MAKE SKILLFUL SAILORS. I originally put these up to help me cope with the challenges in my teaching career. Before I walk out of my art room, I reach up and touch the smaller banner. "Smooth seas don't make skillful sailors," I murmur.

Richard and I walk out to the car together, where Adele is playing her Nintendo DS, held inches from her face, and Matt is bouncing his head to the radio as it blares AC/DC. ". . . She was the best damn woman that I've ever seen . . . you shook me all night long . . ." As I buckle my seatbelt, I think, *Could I have cancer? There's no way. I'm healthy. I eat good food. I exercise and do yoga. I'm the healthiest person I know. I couldn't have cancer. My kids need me . . . my husband couldn't handle parenting these kids without me . . . just look at the kids, there's no way . . . Could I have cancer?* In the car I run with these thoughts and let the music blare and the Nintendo DS be played. Though I'm in a state of shock, I can feel the vitality from letting the inside of the car be crazy, letting my children be a healthy crazy. I remember being young and not so healthy. I remembered being young and just simply crazy.

I usually look forward to the annual Dundee Central School open house. The ten year age gap between my two children means I've been coming to the school's open houses forever. This year it will become my son's alma mater as he graduates in June, just as it was my and my dad's alma mater.

Our family's tradition during open house is to walk the halls and look at all the beautifully framed graduation photos. All these years, I have treasured showing my children these photos at each and every open house. The 1965 graduation pictures of my dad and my godmother—with my dad's handsome, slick Elvis-like hair and my godmother's cat eye glasses—are classic pictures, worth a thousand words.

Gennie and John Salamendra sponsored my Polish family when they first came to the States in 1957. My dad and my uncle John did not speak any English, so they were put in the same classes as the Salamendras' children who were Polish as well and just a bit younger than my dad and Uncle John. Victoria and Anthony spoke both Polish and English, so by placing my father, Stanislaus (Stanley), in Victoria's fourth grade class and Yanushek (John) in Anthony's class, the Salamendra children could translate and tutor my dad and Uncle John while in school. I have always thought my dad was the most amazing person for being able to learn to read, write, and speak English and graduate high school a few short years after he first came to America.

The Salamendra sponsorship also meant that they had to house and employ the Schmidt family for two solid years. They had a large farm and farmhouse and a hired help's home where Grandpa, Grandma, Dad, and Uncle John would live during those years. My grandfather had lied about actually being a farmer on his immigration application papers so that he could immigrate to America. When I was younger, I always thought "lied" was too strong of a word and I now realize that my Polish family would not have known to use a more appropriate word for my grandfather's actions, like "falsehood" or "fib" or "untruth." Anyhow, I thought "lied" was actually more "brave," seeing how he had brought his family across the world for a life in America.

Nonetheless, our families became intertwined and, years later, Victoria and Anthony would eventually become godparents to all of us Schmidt children. Every holiday we'd celebrate our Polish heritage together with traditional Polish foods, and every holiday it took days to prepare all of it. It always involved all the Polish women and lots of port wine. All the pierogi, poppy seed rolls, borscht, horseradish beet spreads, and cabbage dishes they made were enough to feed five Polish clans. The kielbasa, never, ever eaten on Christmas Eve but always at every other Polish event and holiday, and Babka bread, which was made and eaten every Easter morning to celebrate Christ rising, were my favorites. I always asked Genie, who was like a grandma to me, what was in this or that dish and she'd typically answer in her Polish manner while whisking her hand upward. "Mostly eggs," she'd say.

Tonight, the halls of Dundee Central seem more alive to me; getting the call from Beth definitely woke me up. I look closer at my dad's black and white graduation picture, at his beautiful and young eighteen-year-old smile, and wonder how he had coped with his own mother's cancer. All through my younger years I had found it very out of the ordinary that my grandmother was not laid out in a casket in a funeral home. Rather, her wake was in her own living room.

Dad and Uncle John continued to process this traumatic family experience into their adulthood. When I was little, I would ask them how they slept with a dead body in their living room. My uncle would always say the same thing: "Not very damn good." My dad, on the other hand, would try to explain in a developmentally appropriate way, saying that they laid Grandma out in her living room because that was how they did it in Poland when Grandpa was a young boy. He explained that Grandpa was born in 1898 and still did things like they did in "the old country." Grandma died first, of an invasive breast cancer in 1961. She was only forty-seven years old, while my dad was only sixteen and my uncle John was eleven.

I continue to look thoughtfully at my dad's graduation picture. I'm mesmerized by his slicked-back hair, dark eyes, and apparent maturity. Usually I take all of this reminiscing for granted but tonight I sense something more. I notice how my dad looks much more grown-up than he actually should be. I see a deep trauma in his eyes and I momentarily connect as I remember the pain I felt when I lost him when I was just nineteen years old. I'm still staring into that framed glass when Adele tugs on my coat.

"Come on, Mom, let's go to my art room," she says with a smile.

I take one last glance at the picture, seeing my reflection in the glass, and then close my eyes. "I miss my daddy," I whisper quietly. Then I open my eyes and give my daughter a warm smile.

"Sure, honey, show me the way," I say to her.

We wander through the halls of the school. I feel a sense of pride as my daughter skips excitedly down the hallway saying hey to all of her eight-year-old friends. Tonight, my emotional wounds have been opened by the phone call and now life feels uncertain. This uncertainty manifests itself as a feeling of being awake, aware, and compassionate. I smile at everyone, hoping they feel that power in my smile. This is life and we are here in this one body for this one short time. I've learned too many times that we can be whisked away in the blink of an eye; taken away by cancer and taken away by human suffering. I realize that the one good thing to come from my unexpected phone call is that I want to be even more compassionate towards all people. Life has a way of being difficult enough.

~ ~ ~

My dad first got sick in the summer of 1987.

It was an extremely warm June midweek morning. I was living in a downstairs apartment just down the street from my parents. My dad typically popped in sporadically in the morning, afternoon, or evening. In fact, I never knew when he would pop in. He would come on his bike and make sure I was not doing anything I shouldn't have been doing, like having young men over, drinking alcoholic beverages, or doing anything else he didn't approve of.

My dad was doing this because I was only nineteen years old. I had married on a crazy, quirky weekend in front of the justice of the peace at only eighteen years old. I married a boy I dated in my senior year of high school. He wasn't the type of boy my dad really wanted for me. This boyfriend liked to stay out late, drink, and do all the things my parents would never approve of. It was a quick and commotion-filled eight-month marriage. And, if that wasn't enough to piss off and worry my parents to death, I got pregnant right away, carried the baby for nearly five months, lost the baby, and kicked the guy out of our shared apartment. Now I was living on my own, healing my body, and looking for a job.

I lost my baby by some rare, weird fluke. My mom took me to get an ultrasound because the doctors still hadn't heard a heartbeat even though I was nearly twenty weeks pregnant. The doctors were trying to figure this out and began throwing around the term "molar pregnancy," a very rare condition that only occurs in one out of every one thousand pregnancies. A molar pregnancy is a benign growth that grows uncontrollably in the uterus and looks somewhat like grapes. I had to undergo an operation where they dilated my cervix and surgically removed the mass. But in 1987 the doctors didn't really encourage one to grieve the fact that one had lost a baby. Back then, the doctors just shared that their operation was successful; the emotional support to cope with such a loss was never given.

I, however, had always instinctively known that it was necessary to grieve. I went into the hospital bathroom in the middle of the night on my one overnight stay after the procedure, and cried. I looked into the mirror at my tears and then looked up towards heaven. "I was going to name you Jessica." I cried, bent over, and held the sadness in my gut. I looked back in the mirror and wiped my tears. "I name you Jessica." I simultaneously cried and smiled as I thanked my baby for her help in getting me out of the unhealthy relationship I didn't want to be in. I prayed and asked Jessica to watch over any future children I would have. I felt at peace.

Losing a baby at nearly nineteen with someone that I really didn't want to be with anyhow also meant something else to me: "Wow, the universe is now giving me a second chance. I'm going to separate from him. This strife-filled relationship is not what I want. I'm going to get a job, a car, and live life the way I want to live it." I didn't know how I was going to do these things, but I had strong faith and knew my life was unfolding the way it was supposed to unfold.

Once I was home from the hospital, my dad began showing up on his coffee breaks. He would give one knock on my side apartment door and walk right in, opening my refrigerator and cupboards to make sure I had enough food. He would sometimes sit at the kitchen table with me and we would talk about his new job at the disposal company.

I liked sitting with him at the kitchen table, cracking hazelnuts and answering his computer questions. I felt smart, helping the kindest and best man I knew. I did notice that I felt sorry for him. I was sad that he seemed unusually and extremely frustrated with his computer work at his job. He continually told me that his boss wanted him to master the computer for record management and program making. I tried to shrug off his anxiety by thinking, *Well, my dad was born in 1945, you can't expect him to know much about computers.* Since beginning his new job at the disposal company, every pop-in visit ended with me reassuring him.

"Don't worry, Dad, you'll get it. I'll stop by and help you later." My dad always gave me a kiss on my cheek before saying "I love you, Poopaa."

Then, on that Wednesday morning of June 10, 1987, my dad didn't come to my house for his coffee break. Nor did he show for work. Rather, he walked out of his home, wandered off, and ended up on a quiet country road, literally staring at the sun. A woman who knew him was walking her dog. She saw him and said, "Hi Stan!" Everyone in this small town knew everyone! But she quickly realized he was acting unusual because he didn't respond to her at all. Instead, he focused on her dog, who was barking at him. He bent down as if he was going to pick up the dog by its neck, then stopped himself and continued walking aimlessly down the dirt road. The woman, alarmed by his odd behavior, quickly walked her dog home and called the police out of concern for my dad.

Meanwhile, my dad's boss, Dick, came knocking on my door.

"Have you seen your father?" he had asked me.

I wanted to spit in his face and answer with something like "Get the hell off my doorstep! If you'd stop riding his ass about learning the computer and managing your crappy trash disposal company maybe he wouldn't be acting so stressed out all the time." Instead I replied with a shocked tone because my dad always went to work.

"Why, he's not at work?"

Seeing that I honestly didn't know where my father was, he quickly turned his back and walked towards his brand-new red Chevy truck.

"If you see him, just tell him I'm looking for him," he yelled, waving his hand in the air.

I knew my dad had been acting odd for a few months, stressed out from his new job as manager. A few months before, he had come to me not knowing what to do when two of his garbage men came into the office smelling like they had just put out a marijuana joint, their eyes red and hazy.

"Dad, they're garbage men! Let it go!" I had advised him with my usual nineteen-year-old wisdom.

My dad hadn't been sleeping though and he certainly was not letting anything go. Within an hour of Dick's knock on my door, my mom called from the local hospital saying that Dad had been picked up on a back road by the police because he was "acting weird."

I took in everything Mom said and then practically hung up the phone on her. I quickly threw on the previous day's clothes that were still lying on my bedroom floor and fast-pulled my hair back into a pony-tail. I grabbed my purse, a bottle of cola from the fridge, my cigarettes from the counter, and ran to my blue '79 Ford Pinto. I hurled my things onto the passenger seat and slammed the car door. As I started the car, I noticed that I hadn't even shut my apartment door and that the screen door was flapping. But I didn't care about anything but my dad. I put the car in reverse and sped down Hollister Street and then onto Route 14A, off to Penn Yan. I lit a cigarette with my car lighter and pressed on the gas pedal, making it a seventy-five-mile-per-hour race to the hospital. I knew I could be at the local hospital in fifteen minutes. My thoughts rushed with each smoky inhalation: *What the hell is going on?*

When I got to the hospital, I saw my mom standing next to a police car and talking to four officers. The parking lot was hot from the humid weather and steamy pavement. I smashed my second cig-arette of the short trip into the cement and rushed over to where they were. The back doors of the car were open and I saw my dad lying face down on the floor with shackles around his ankles and his hands cuffed behind his back. He was repeating letters of the alphabet: "M, m, m, m, m, m . . ."

"Oh my God! What the hell is going on?" I pushed through my mom and the officers and went directly to the back seat. "Dad, it's okay, I'm here . . . it's me, Poopaa!" I said to him as I rubbed his back. He stopped repeating letters for a moment, and I was sure it was because he heard my voice and the childhood name he always called me. His body was warm and he was sweating pro-fusely. I looked up with the best pissed off look anyone could ever have. I was furious at the officers and my mom, furious at them for standing around talking rather than consoling my dad. Something was obviously wrong with him.

"Honey, they're going to take your dad to Willard Psychiatric Center," my mom said calmly while looking directly at me. "They couldn't find anything physically wrong with him at this hospital and they need to take him to the psychiatric ward for an evaluation."

I knew the look my mom was giving me. Her fixed stare said, *Don't make a scene in front of these nice officers or so help me God.*

I gave her back my angry gawk, hoping she would read my mind too. My mind was screaming *Who the hell are you? Talking so nicely and calmly in front of the police when Dad is lying in shackles in their car?*

Instead of screaming, I answered somewhat respectfully. "What the hell is going on? Dad is not crazy! He's just stressed out from his job."

An officer calmly touched my shoulder and I quickly pulled away from his touch.

"Your father was found wandering on a back road this morning," he said to me. "He had become confrontational with a woman's dog and did not respond to her." He told me everything in a police-like reporting manner. I listened to the droning of his voice and pictured it all in my head, then lit up another cigarette. The police officer told me I could follow him over to the psychiatric ward. It was on the other side of the lake.

Of course, going into the local supermarket after this incident was traumatic in and of itself. The whispers—"That's her, her dad went crazy"—seemed to follow me everywhere in town. One young man, Al, actually stopped me in the grocery store to sincerely ask how my dad was doing, in a caring and non-judgmental manner. I could hardly believe that someone was talking directly to me about my dad. Every other acquaintance I ran into never straightforwardly spoke to me about it. Rather, they just whispered after I had walked by.

I thought the whole event regarding my dad must have been traumatic for this quiet, small town that shut down all business on Sundays. But every time I saw Al, he was not traumatized by the event. He was considerate and caring. I had intellectual and thoughtful conversations about my dad with Al. It seemed he was the only one that cared and wasn't afraid to talk about it with me. I eventually invited Al over to my apartment and we fell in love. I took him on visits to see my dad. Since then, I've always thought it took a real kind and good man to go to a psychiatric ward to meet a girlfriend's father for the first time. I needed a kind man, especially when it came to visiting my dad in the psychiatric ward.

My father stayed at this psychiatric center for the next three months because of having been involuntarily committed.

When anyone was involuntarily committed to a psychiatric ward, it was a long process to get out; you couldn't simply "check yourself out." You had to earn your way out with weekend visits and good behavior. My dad would have ongoing electroshock therapy in a tightly locked security ward and be pumped up daily with a drug called Thorazine. Doctors prescribed it to those patients who suffered a loss of their normal personality and to those who had combative and explosive behaviors. The combination of shock therapy and the medicine took my dad way past just unusual anxiety. To me, he appeared sedated and nuttier than ever. He walked around with a shuffle, like a zombie, unlike the dad that I truly knew. He stayed in the ward until the doctors realized he never went crazy at all but instead had a brain tumor. By then, though, it was too late, as it had metastasized to his lungs and was now everywhere in his body.

3

"Thank God This Is Only an Office Procedure"

October 19, 2009

I take a half day off from work to go have the endometrial biopsy Beth has recommended. I pull into the parking lot and feel irritated by all the changes with this building. This was the place where I gave birth to my daughter in a queen-sized bed with my husband coaching me as my midwife helped deliver our eight-pound, eleven-ounce baby girl, all without any medication. Beth has sent me here because she doesn't perform doctoral procedures—such as biopsies—at her place.

The building used to be a women's center with midwives, HypnoBirthing classes, Lamaze classes, and prenatal yoga. It was everything I stood for, and what once felt sacred now appears more like any other bureaucratic hospital. It still has a home-like feel; however, its environment has been converted into a hospital-like venue. It now has an office or two for a doctor, along with a few procedure rooms. The whole birthing area has been turned into a center for studying sleep disorders.

I handle missing my old women's center by running with my critical thoughts: *Thank God this is only an office procedure.* I dislike being around any type of hospital setting. I have worked very hard in my adult life to transform my past, cigarette-smoking, unfocused young self to a career-bound, healthy yoga guru, mother of two, and happily married woman. I am a grown-up and determined to be a healthy woman. I have labeled myself a "woman's center" type of client, not a patient in a hospital. My judgments of this transformed medical establishment run through my mind.

Once inside, I'm asked to sit in the waiting room. Time hangs, especially since I can hardly connect with this place or with any of the typical medical, young parenting, or travel magazines. I decide to close my eyes and practice my breathing techniques to calm myself.

The nurse appears through the double door, only barely poking herself into the waiting area. I open my eyes and see her white clogs perkily together, ready to march back for the next office procedure. She is standing with perfect posture in her brightly colored linen scrubs and is the perfect picture of the twenty-first-century nurse. She has her to-go coffee mug in one hand, a caffeinated smile, and a clipboard in her other arm.

I feel exhausted just looking at her bouncy energy. I am mostly tired from my exhausting judgmental thoughts; oh, and let's not forget that I have been teaching and caring for eighteen preschoolers for the first half of my day. I give her a tired smile before reluctantly getting up from the comfy couch and walking towards her. She immediately turns and begins her lively stride down the hallway. I follow her perky voice. "We're just going to this procedure room down the hall."

She takes me to the room that used to be the library area when this building was the women's center, turning the antique glass doorknob and holding the door open for me. I immediately remember its specialness from all my prenatal visits when I was pregnant over eight years ago. It was a small and elegant room that had a few comfy chairs and shelves filled with motherhood and birthing picture books. The room had flower-print wallpaper and I remember how I loved the tempered lighting provided by a lamp placed on top of a crocheted doily on an antique table.

I remember sitting in that library and looking through pictures of midwifery books when I was pregnant. Back in 2000 I wanted to have a natural childbirth with no medication. My natural childbirth decision was due in part because in 1990, when I gave birth to my son, I had been given Demerol for my extreme labor pains. I was in labor for over fourteen hours and I was having difficulty pushing my son out, so he had to be pulled out with forceps. He came out lethargic and had a huge bump on the right side of his head. So, when I was pregnant again, I loved looking at the natural childbirth books in the library. I had been determined to go natural and to be present throughout my delivery experience. I had chosen to give birth at this women's center because it reflected my current healthy-yoga-type personality. It was the perfect wholesome place.

I recognize the room right away. The wallpaper and crown molding are still the same. However, the motherhood books are now gone and have been replaced with glass jars filled with gauze and cotton balls. There are also some towels and medical gowns neatly folded on the bottom shelf. The reading lamp and antique table are also gone and there is now a medical exam light and a desk near the window in their place.

Looking around the room at all of its changes, I tell the nurse that I gave birth in this building.

She politely connects. "I hear Beth's women's center is doing well."

I feel my tired self turn more accepting towards this new medical center, happy that the nurse knows my midwife.

"Oh, you know Beth?"

She shakes my hand. "Yes. I'm Leigh, Dr. Daye's nurse."

Throughout our lengthy conversation, I really begin to like Leigh. She is a young, thin woman with traditional, yet stylish nurse scrubs on. She looks cute in them. Her uniform shirt is tied off to one side, almost like a yoga workout top which, of course, I like even more. I begin to feel connected and more comfortable and I open up to share more about myself. She asks me about my family history and continues writing this information down on her clipboard paper. As I tell Leigh about my family history of cancer—my mother, father, both grandmothers, plus others—she pauses and looks up at me as if a light bulb has turned on inside of her. Her eyes appear even bigger.

"We now do genetic testing here, and I think you would qualify!" she shares eagerly.

"What's genetic testing?" I ask.

"Well, we can see if you test positive for a cancer gene, and if you do, then the doors open for you in the insurance world. Sometimes insurance will only offer coverage for, let's say a breast MRI, if there is a problem. Or, they might only cover a colonoscopy if you are over fifty. However, if you test positive for a cancer gene, your insurance would allow you to have these tests at a younger age. You wouldn't have to wait until you get cancer for the insurance to cover these procedures. You can keep a more comprehensive surveillance on yourself so you don't get cancer. Or if you do get cancer, you catch it real early."

Leigh says this enthusiastically—almost in one, long breath—and I'm surprised by it all.

"Why doesn't everyone get tested then?" I ask her.

Her eyes open up as wide as they can. "Well, you have to qualify, and the two tests that I want the doctor to give you are both over three thousand dollars each. However, if you qualify, these tests won't cost anything to you." She pauses for a moment and nods her head to see if I understand everything she is telling me.

"How do I qualify?" I ask.

She looks down at the history she's already recorded on her clipboard. "I think you already do. You have a long family history of cancer and you've had an abnormal pap smear. Let's talk to the doctor when he comes in."

Leigh instructs me to go ahead and sit on the exam table, telling me that, because I have a skirt on, it won't be necessary to put on a hospital gown. I climb up on the table and mull over everything Leigh has just shared. My mind doesn't see any issue with this new genetic test. It only sees proactive involvement at its highest level, and proactive has always been my middle name, so why wouldn't anyone in their right mind do this? I can't think of one reason *not* to be tested.

Leigh is flipping through her paperwork when Dr. Dayes gives one knock and walks into the room with a cane. He is a heavy-set, older man with glasses, and sweat is coming down on either side of his face. He gives me a nod and a brief hello as he slowly sits down at the desk. His breathing seems heavy, probably because of the extra weight he is carrying. I know from living in the small Finger Lakes region that he lost his wife to breast cancer last year. I also assume that this is probably part of the reason why he hasn't retired yet. His irritable disposition tells me it has been a long day for him and he just wants to get this last procedure of the day over with. His young animated nurse thankfully serves as a counterbalance to his crankiness.

Leigh runs my history by him as if I'm not in the room, pointing to all the history she has recorded for him. ". . . and I think she qualifies for genetic testing too."

He signs everything she puts in front of him and then tiredly turns to me.

"Okay, let's have a look and then we'll let Leigh draw your blood."

I don't feel comfortable with his tired demeanor. I feel like I am just another patient, just another number, and just another procedure. I don't want this feeling and I don't want this medical atmosphere, so I spontaneously pull out some quick knowledge I have about Dr. Dayes. I hope that, in doing so, it will provide for a more personal space. I want Dr. Dayes to see me for the healthy person I am. I want to feel better before getting any painful procedure done. My gut tells me to speak up, so I decide to try and get him to connect with me using what quick information I can share about his career and interests.

I tighten my knees together.

"I saw you on *The Today Show* this past summer promoting home birthing," I blurt out.

My comment elicits a smile from Dr. Hayes.

"Yeah, I'm still taking flak for that interview," he says with a grin.

I have my list of questions prepared and ready, everything from the possible hysterectomy to other cancer questions. As I start to ask him the questions, he interrupts me.

"Look, you're premenopausal. Irregular pap smears are normal at your age. I can tell, just by looking at you, that it's probably just a mild dysplasia."

I'm shocked. "You can tell by looking at me? Beth says the HPV is HPV 53, which is a high risk one." I have mixed feelings here because he is saying that I look healthy, which is kind of a compliment, but on the other hand I know, deep in my heart, that my healthy self can't be totally immune to cancer. I trust my gut again, especially given my family's history.

"Look, I've been doing this a long time, over thirty-five years, and an abnormal pap smear at your age is normal." As he lays me back on the table, he continues demonstrating his medical knowledge. "Your HPV 53 is not one of the squirrelly whirly HPVs, like HPV 16 or 18. So, now let's have a look."

Leigh is continuously sugarcoating all of his sourness.

"Dr. Dayes took care of a female issue I was having a few years back. I thank God for his expertise," she says as she puts my feet in the stirrups.

Since I actually like Leigh, I decide to talk more with her and let Dr. Dayes chime in when he feels the need to trump our conversation with some of his medical knowledge.

Dr. Dayes has a small lamp he wears around his head. As he inserts the metal speculum into my vagina, I tense up. He tells me to relax and I take a deep breath. He explains that he is going to do the endocervical biopsy first and tells Leigh that he is biopsying at twelve, two, and seven o'clock on my cervix. I feel every little piece being ripped from my cervix and I am proud of myself for breathing deeply. I also make ongoing jokes about how much pain I've had to go through in this building, first with childbirth and now this. Then he explains that for the endometrial biopsy he will be taking a needle and going up through my cervix and into the uterus for the tissue. I squeeze Leigh's hand as he performs this part of the procedure. I look in her eyes. "My God!"

She wipes my hair to the side. "We're almost finished."

When we are done, Dr. Dayes and Leigh help me sit up, keeping the white hospital sheet over my work dress, which I never took off.

Dr. Dayes taps my knee and consoles me. "Don't worry! This is nothing, just mild dysplasia."

"How can you be sure?" I ask, wiping away a few tears from the painful biopsy.

"Look, what is your favorite restaurant?" he responds.

"Jerlando's, in Watkins Glen," I say, slightly confused.

He puts his hands on both of my knees and looks directly into my eyes. "If this is cancer, I will buy you dinner every day for a whole year. I just know."

I look down and smile, wondering why it is that I now seem to like Dr. Dayes. I realize that he reminds me of my dysfunctional, gambling Polish family. His ethnicity is strong. He is who he is, and he does what he does. He never questions his actions, only honors them, making them a part of his everyday self. I like this confidence.

As Dr. Dayes leaves the procedure room, he gives me a nod. "Have a good evening," he says.

I notice that it's now dark outside and that the receptionist has shut off most of the lights in the building.

Leigh draws my blood. "Now these genetic tests take time, so let's set a follow-up in a week and a half. The blood work should be back by then and we'll have your results from the biopsies too. Also, if you feel any pain this evening, just take some Ibuprofen." She puts gauze in the crook of my arm and places a piece of tape over it. "Call if you need anything."

I smile sadly with pain and tell her I'm going home to have a glass of wine and confess that I'm calling in sick tomorrow.

"That's a good idea," she says warmly.

On the way home, I call Richard, who also supports my decision to call in sick, and I tell him I'll be home shortly.

The drive home is painful. I feel uncomfortable sitting upright and feel a strong pressure below my abdomen. I just want to be home, reclining in my sofa with a glass of red wine in my hand. I take deep breaths and turn on the radio to distract myself. Delilah is on, one of my favorite syndicated radio shows, and I listen to some of the sappiest love songs ever made. I usually listen to her with an amused disposition; however, tonight she is discussing some heart-wrenching health issue with a woman and how much that woman loves the man who is taking care of her, emotionally and physically. Delilah plays a sentimental song to help the woman heal her way back to health and back to her old self again. Tonight, I listen to her with an aware disposition and set aside my judgments. I take her love seriously. I cry as I listen to the woman's touching story and then sing along to Van Morrison's "Have I Told You Lately That I Love You?" I pull into my driveway and wipe away my tears. I take another deep breath, open the car door, and slowly shift my legs outward to exit the car.

I walk stiffly into my house and when I get in my kitchen, I feel this amazing sense of relief to be home. I hear Matt playing his guitar in his bedroom and I know it's Adele's bath time. The routine of my life brings me such contentment and comfort. The biopsies, this small trauma of life, helps me to be thankful for this routine. I walk around uncomfortably and work to get my mind at ease before calling in sick tomorrow.

Once I call in, I can feel my body relax a bit more. I pour a glass of wine, take an Ibuprofen, and sit in the recliner with my feet up. I close my eyes and breathe in the memory of my mom and her lifestyle. She would never have drunk a glass of wine and taken an Ibuprofen. Her lifestyle was more like vodka and Valium.

Mom's purse was always filled with prescription bottles. If anyone within an arm's length said they had a cough or a sore throat, my mom would pull something from her heavy, pill-laden purse. "Here, take this." I think her doctor, Dr. Muck, secretly had a crush on her. Either that or he was easily amused by her. He gave her anything she asked for. She had been able to balance most of the prescriptions with Old Milwaukee her whole life, but it went way out of control when my dad was in the psychiatric hospital.

During that time, my brother, uncle, and I were becoming quite the Euchre card players with the rest of the patients at the Willard

Psychiatric Center. Many of the patients lit up when they saw us come through the locked doors and into their activity room. The security guard was always glad to see us as well and he shared that most of their patients didn't get many visitors. He added that he also liked our interaction with the Willard staff members.

Dad would greet us and we'd all gather around the large, wooden dining table in the middle of the activity room. Rose, an older homeless patient, always crocheted and asked questions about our family. I realized later that she wasn't crazy, just homeless. Of course, there were crazy people there, like the woman who sat cross-legged on the floor with headphones on and rocked back and forth. I had a habit of staring at her, wondering if her brain hurt from all that flopping around and loud music, until I noticed that her headphones weren't even plugged into a music player. She looked pale and distant and very crazy. I felt sad and wondered what had happened for her to act this way.

There was also a man that wore white socks and a too small, dark polyester suit. He looked like a nerdy Charles Manson, always standing and looking out the window. He made me a little nervous because he never responded to my "Hi there! How are you today?" Rather, he'd angle his head and look at me with empty eyes. I felt sad for him too and wondered if he felt loved. The security guard would try and joke with him by putting both of his hands on the man's shoulders.

"Come on, Henry, don't you see that the pretty gal is asking how you are today?" he'd say, giving me a wink.

Every time the security guard took us through the locked doors and into the activity room, my brother Ben, Uncle John, and I would joke with him while signing our names on the arrivals' sheet.

"Now, you're going to let us back through when we're ready to leave, right?" Uncle John would ask. He always had a small fear that they wouldn't let us leave, partly because he often smoked a tiny pin joint before entering the building and was therefore paranoid. Since he had returned from Vietnam, he had always been very good at letting his paranoid behavior take over anyhow.

Sometimes my mom would already be signed in and "visiting" with my dad by the time we arrived, smoking cigarettes and laughing with Rose and the other patients. I could always tell by her slurry words that she'd been taking more than her usual Valium.

Dad generally looked numb. Ben, Uncle John, and I would just sit down and ignore Mom's highness and eventually pull out the deck of cards we brought along for the day.

Dad always looked forward to our arrival. He'd kiss my cheek. "I missed you, Poopaa!" he'd say. I still noticed his Thorazine shuffle as he walked around the activity room like a stiff robot. I hated seeing him like this and I always felt sad every time I arrived. My sadness ran deep into my heart because Dad had always been the strong one, the bread winner, the straight-laced, big bicep push-up guy, the one who carried Mom to bed when she drank too much.

As my mother smoked and laughed with the psychiatric patients and my dad shuffled around the activity room, I'd feel the need, in the pit of my stomach, to blame someone for all of this. I had a deep need to blame my mom for allowing the police to bring Dad here. I also blamed my dad's boss, Dick, for continually nagging my dad to master that lousy computer of his. I really did hate my dad being in this hellhole but I showed up daily with my cards. I took the forty-five minute drive over on one side of Seneca Lake and traveled another forty-five minutes to come back on the other side of it. "Do you have to go already?" Dad would say every time when it was time for us to leave. I hated leaving him there but I always assured him that he would be able to come home for a weekend visit soon and that we'd play cards then too. I yearned to be back to normal, back to the normal amount of Valium pills for Mom, the normal amount of booze and pot for my uncle, and normal card playing around my family's kitchen table.

4

The Twists and Turns of Waiting

Even though Leigh told me the test results would take a week and a half to come back and Dr. Dayes told me basically not to worry about these abnormal pap results—that it's simply mild dysplasia—my imaginative mind runs with all the worse case scenarios. I'm not new to this type of thinking, which I call "What if" thoughts.

For the most part, I usually envision the same thoughts in my mind. The "What if I have cancer?" scene always includes me with no hair, no eyebrows, no eyelashes, bone thin, and videotaping myself to give my kids a last offering of advice that they probably won't take anyhow. The "What if I can't work anymore?" scene always includes my family having to sell our home, our cars, our worldly possessions of . . . well, we actually don't have any travel souvenirs. Even if we did, we wouldn't have them anymore. The scene includes my family not having two nickels to rub together. The "What if I lose my home?" scene always follows the "What if I can't work anymore?" scenario. I envision moving in with some family member with all of our cardboard boxes filled with trinkets and all of our trivial objects.

Next, the "What if my children are traumatized?" scene always includes, once again, me videotaping my advice to my children that they won't take, actually stating this fact in the video, and then providing them the phone number of some good counselor for when they might need it later in life. The "What if I lose all my possessions?" scene usually involves me sitting in an empty room with my hairless head between my bony knees, crying pathetically over some knickknacks and CorningWare dishes. Now the last two, "What if I die?" and "What if Richard can't take care of the kids?" always involve me privately touching base with one of my good friends to make sure someone will be available to take over caring for my family: braiding Adele's hair, fixing some good meals, and hosting every holiday get together. She would need to be Richard's companion, and I'd prefer someone in the Dundee School district so my children wouldn't get overly traumatized by a move (in addition to me dying). Whew! It truly is going to be a long week and a half waiting for these results.

For the last ten years, I've been practicing meditation and yoga to counter these tiring and ludicrous thought patterns of mine. I've been doing so much yoga that I've actually become certified as a sport toga instructor. My new, higher self became aware of how to take life back from unnecessary "What If" thoughts through these two activities.

It still takes a lot of work though. All of the thoughts that I can run with have to be countered each time with "If you have cancer, then you will deal with it, just like your parents dealt with their cancer. You don't have any results yet, so breathe. All is well." The old thought will argue more, and my new self will oppose and answer wisely. It is during this time that I realize I never truly got rid of my old self. I never transformed totally. Rather, I have only learned how to calm down my old thoughts.

The night before my appointment, I drink some valerian root tea just as I get ready for bed. I have kissed the kids goodnight and do not anticipate a very good night's sleep with all the "What ifs" pounding in my mind. I sit in bed holding my favorite blue ceramic mug that I made years ago in an art class. As I hold the warm tea mug in both of my hands, I look around at all my artwork hanging in my bedroom. In the nineties, I went through a phase of creating paintings with road signs as the subject. I thought road signs portrayed powerful messages in my art. To the left of me is a painting I made back in 1997. It is a large acrylic painting, thirty by thirty-six inches, of an outdoor scene with a road that comes to a T. This particular painting has, as its focal point, a big yellow road sign with black arrows pointing to the left and to the right. Obviously, any driver coming to a sign like the one in my painting would have to make a decision—do you turn left or right? I can see, through the mirror hanging on the wall in front of me, another large painting of a road sign I created back in 1996. That road sign is a warning to slow down because you are approaching a sharp corner. There are beautiful lilacs in that painting; the message I meant to convey was to slow down and smell the flowers.

I become aware of my breathing, and I calm my heart and my mind with "Slow down. All is well. All is perfectly unfolding." I now feel very sleepy and I place my empty tea mug on my nightstand and curl up on my side in a fetal position. My husband comes in and kisses me goodnight and says he is heading downstairs to watch some hockey. I smile and give him a tired "Okay." I close my eyes and feel gratitude drift through my body; for my wonderful family, comfy queen-sized bed, cozy pillow, and my inspirational road-sign paintings. I am thankful for the valerian root tea. I wake up appreciating the much needed good night's sleep and with a clear mind ready to take on anything that life hands me.

❧ ❧ ❧

October 28, 2009
The day of my appointment, I arrive at Dr. Daye's office after work. It's a late-day appointment, and from the moment I step into the building I sense that everyone knows something that I don't. The receptionist doesn't even ask me for my name.

"Have a seat, Angela. Leigh will be right with you."

I sit in the waiting room and hear the receptionist walk directly upstairs. Within moments, Leigh follows her back downstairs and into the waiting room.

"Hi Angela, come right back."

We walk back to the same procedure room from a week and a half ago, Leigh making only small talk with me and not making any real eye contact.

"The weather is beautiful today. I just love fall."

I agree, feeling slightly irritated by the small talk. "Yes, fall is a beautiful time of year."

The room looks the same, however there is now an extra wooden chair placed to one side. The three wooden chairs are in a sort of circle, ready for a meeting to discuss something important. This is another clue that something could be wrong.

"Angela, have a seat. Dr. Dayes will be right with you." Leigh points to the far wooden chair, which obviously appears to be "the patient's chair."

I sit down and Leigh fidgets with some papers and keeps the small talk going. "School is going good?"

I really just want to get my results and I'm hoping Leigh will shed some light on them. "It's fine!" I answer, then come right out and ask, "How did all my tests come back?" I ask this knowing I won't get any definitive answers since Leigh is the nurse. But I know I can at least get part of an answer from her body language.

Leigh doesn't look at me in my eyes as she answers. "Dr. Dayes is going to go over *everything* with you."

Her answer tells me *everything* means *something* is wrong. One of the gifts I received by growing up as the oldest girl in an alcoholic home is that I'm an extremely sensitive person. I can pick up on the slightest negative energy and I know when something is even a little wrong. I have also fine-tuned my spiritual ability to feel that intense energy in the air. Sometimes I cannot clearly articulate what the energy is about, but I'm always keenly aware of its presence. When I combine the lack of eye contact, the anxious body language, her word choice of *everything,* and the intense energy in the air, it all equates to something being definitely wrong.

Leigh places a pen on top of my file and smiles as she says she will be right back with the doctor. As she leaves the procedure room, I close my eyes and take a deep breath. In that moment, I feel this amazing atmospheric and spiritual energy in the room. I know I am surrounded by Mom's, Dad's, and Grandmother's spirits. The energy makes me feel safe and powerful. I definitely know that there is something wrong in this human world. But their spirits are here with me now to give me the message that everything is perfectly alright too. I close my eyes again and whisper "thank you" out loud to them for this reassurance.

I take several more deep breaths and hear Leigh and Dr. Dayes coming down the hall. Once again, Dr. Dayes enters the room out of breath and with sweat running down the side of his face. He gives me a "Good afternoon!" and I politely smile and nod at his gesture. I'm sometimes amazed that people aren't aware of the powerful spiritual energy that is around them.

Leigh hands him my paperwork as he sits in one of the wooden chairs by the desk. Leigh sits properly in the other wooden chair, bouncing her crossed leg and ready to help the doctor with his curt bedside manner. Dr. Dayes opens my file and reviews it. I put my elbows on my knees, lean in, and look directly at him, ready to take on every word he has to say, every diagnosis he has to give. He looks at Leigh, then back at me.

"You have tested positive for BRCA1, the hereditary breast and ovarian cancer gene. This is very rare and we are going to do every possible test to see if you have cancer anywhere in your body."

My jaw drops. "Do you think I have cancer?"

Dr. Dayes fixes his glasses. "Listen, these tests are all very new to this office."

Once again, being the sensitive person that I am to body language and voice tones, I feel his response really means "I'm not sure!"

"You're not sure if I have cancer. What was this genetic test for, then?" I ask.

"These are thorough tests and there can be no error with them," he responds. "You tested positive for carrying a hereditary breast and ovarian cancer gene. We've only had one other woman test positive, but it was for BRCA2. You are the first here to test positive for BRCA1, so I'm going to send you down to the hospital right now for a CA125 blood test and," pointing at me he adds, "if that comes back elevated I'm going to put you in the hospital tomorrow and do an emergency TAH/BSO."

"A *what?*" I shriek.

"A TAH/BSO: Total Abdominal Hysterectomy with a Bilateral Salpingo-Oophorectomy," he says quickly.

I now feel somewhat in safe hands with Dr. Dayes in control of this situation; however, I feel insecure and scared of the unknown. He truly doesn't know whether I have cancer, and I certainly don't know either.

I start to get weepy-eyed. "An emergency hysterectomy?"

He hands me the paper from the blood test, this time pointing and shaking his finger at me like a stern father might do.

"Do not wait on this! You should also have a mastectomy."

I look at the paper he hands me. It reads, "HBOC 5385insC gene positive."

He points to Leigh and speaks in a clear, strong voice.

"I want a transvaginal ultrasound ordered, followed by an abdominal-pelvic CAT scan. Order an upper MRI and a colonoscopy as well." He looks at me and adds, "We're going to see if you have cancer anywhere in your body."

Leigh is quickly writing down everything he says and I hand him back the paper.

"Don't wait on this," Dr. Dayes says again. "Now go directly to the hospital lab before they close."

I gather up my purse and jacket and head down to the lab. I can hear him telling Leigh to call the lab and make sure they don't close. He wants me to have this CA125 blood test done immediately.

By the time I'm leaving the hospital, it's dark outside and approaching early evening. I feel scared and can feel my heart pounding as I rush to my car. I know I should call Richard to tell him I'll be late for dinner but my mind is surprisingly numb. *Holy Jesus, what just happened?* I think to myself. *Holy Mother!* I feel like I need to only take care of myself right now. I feel powerless because the only thing I can do to take care of myself is get some blood work drawn and then wait. I'm shocked by today's test results and wonder just how much more shocked I could ever get from this point on.

5

Testing for My Legacy

The next day my "What if" thoughts kick into high gear. Although I perform every relaxation technique there is—warm baths, meditation, apply lavender lotion, yoga with nature sounds, yoga in silence, yoga with a water fountain—my "What if's" are flowing into my mind every few moments. The one good thing about being in the "What if" zone is that I am also continually asking myself, "Well, *what if* I do have cancer? Then how do I want to live?" I always answer myself with the same response: "Live with compassion."

I've noticed that when I live with compassion towards all people and things, I feel very awake to life. When I am awake to life, I'm more in the moment. When I'm more in the moment, I feel more joy in my heart.

My smile stays with me and I appreciate everything around me more than ever. I love my children, my job, my husband, my life. I love life! I love life and want my life more than ever. So when Leigh calls me at work and asks to be connected to my room, I hold my breath as she shares the results: "Your CA125 blood test came back normal. This is good news."

I breathe and cry. "Oh my God, thank God. I was preparing myself to have this emergency hysterectomy tomorrow."

"Now, we need to make sure you don't have cancer anywhere else," says Leigh. "So we are going to keep all the upcoming tests. I've scheduled them for November 10, beginning at one thirty in the afternoon."

I take out the little diary that I've begun to carry with me in my pocket and write down everything Leigh tells me. Leigh is like a beautiful hummingbird and flutters it all out in one breath.

"We're sending you to Arnot Hospital where you can have everything done at one place. Now, at one thirty you're going to have a transvaginal ultrasound. Then you'll go directly to radiology where you will drink half a smoothie at two fifteen. Drink the other half at three fifteen. The smoothie is no big deal; it's so they can see what is going on inside you. You'll then have your upper MRI at three thirty followed by an abdominal-pelvic CAT scan at four."

"I can do this all in one day?"

She tries to reassure me. "Angela, this is the best thing. Yes! But I couldn't get you in for a colonoscopy until November 25."

I take a deep breath and then say, "Not to take away from Dr. Daye's professional opinion, but I would like to have a few other opinions on what Dr. Dayes is recommending me to do. I mean, asking me to have a total hysterectomy and a total mastectomy when I'm only forty-one years old is a lot. Don't you agree?"

Leigh continues with her reassurances. "Dr. Dayes wouldn't take that personally. Don't worry! I'd do the same thing if I were in your shoes. I'm going to get some numbers for you to get two or three opinions. This is the first time we have had a positive BRCA1 patient," she adds eagerly. "So this is all new to us as well. I'll call you tomorrow with those names."

I'm excited that my CA125 came back normal, less than 6.1 according to Leigh. The CA125 (Cancer Antigen 125) is a protein that is produced in cancer cells. The normal range of CA125 in blood serum levels are 0–35. Dr. Dayes wants my CA125 blood test to be less than 20, so my number falls well within the "okay" range.

Leigh tells me that if it had been elevated above 21, Dr. Dayes would have wanted to operate right away. This is because I would have had two strikes against me in regards to ovarian cancer. We know that I've already tested positive for the hereditary breast and ovarian cancer gene (HBOC). Since my CA125 level is within normal limits— and therefore only have one strike—I am free from emergency surgeries at this time. I finish writing down the information she gives me and then put my pocket diary away.

Although I don't know everything about all these cancer tests, my friend Bill, who died of cancer a few years back, always told me that cancer is "all about the numbers." He told me this when I gave him a hug one day and told him he looked fabulous. He then reluctantly shared that his blood test numbers didn't lie and that his cancer was progressing. I sadly asked him how this could be when he looked so great. He shrugged, shook his head, and looked down. "Cancer is all about the numbers."

My hand is still on the phone receiver and I am immediately frozen in gratitude for Leigh's news. I take a deep breath and can feel Bill's feisty voice in my heart: "Angela, your numbers are frickin' good."

I head back to my students who are with my assistant and are now playing in their learning centers, I murmur to myself, "My numbers are good!"

～ ～ ～

November 7, 2009
Today is my daughter's party. Her actual birthday isn't until Monday, but who wants to have a birthday on a Monday? So, we book the local youth center in Dundee where all of her nine-year-old friends can play pool, foosball, ping-pong, and eat pizza and cheese puffs. I want this to be the best birthday ever for her. *What if this is the last birthday party of hers that I ever see?*

I have put on my youthful blue jeans and gray hooded sweatshirt and braid my hair into two braids. I look in the mirror at myself and think how cute I look, and then I pretend to be nine years old as I run into Adele's bedroom. I dance around her room and wake her up.

"Come on, it's a special day today and I want to be the first one at the birthday party, at the birthday party," I say, and as Adele opens her eyes to look at me, I put my hands on my hips and bump them back and forth and finish with "at the birthday party, at the birthday party."

Adele smiles and pretends not to like me, something that has started only recently. I hate the fact that the "tweenage" years are starting earlier than they did with my son. She hides her head under the blankets so I can't see her smiling. The only thing I like about this limbotime, when I don't actually know what is going on within my body, is that I continually keep thinking, *What the heck, dance like there is no tomorrow.* I secretly hope that when all of this is said and done, and if I don't have cancer, I want to have more fun in my life and not take things—life—so damn seriously all the time. This serious thinking on life has been an issue I've been working on virtually all of my adult life, and limboland is changing me.

Throughout the day, I cheerfully pile things for the party on the island in our kitchen. It starts off with a large picnic basket full of junk food, sour cream chips, ruffled chips, barbeque chips, cheese puff balls, cheese puff twists, cheese puff sticks, and several types of cookies. Then I add another picnic basket to the island and begin including Happy Birthday napkins, Happy Birthday plates, Happy Birthday banners, candles, streamers, and Happy Birthday paper cups. The cake is beautiful, and I set it to the side knowing I want Adele to carry it on her lap on the way to the party. I truly want her to never forget this party, especially in the event that this is the last I get to celebrate with her.

Later, I find a larger box and put some music CDs and my CD player in it. I find some yarn and hope I can teach this new digital generation a childhood game that I used to play for hours on end: cat's cradle. Every so often, after playing with her LEGOs, Adele comes into the kitchen to show me the newest contraption she's just completed and to ask me if it is time to go yet. Each time she asks, I tease her by doing the same little dance. I smile and put my hands on my hips and bump them to the two words I say: "Not yet."

She turns away every time smiling and rolling her eyes, pretending not to like my good attitude. I actually let her get away with the eye rolling, especially since she is getting used to my new lighthearted demeanor. Limboland has put me in a space of loving myself and every moment.

The pile keeps getting bigger and when Richard wakes up from his nap, I point to the stack and ask him if he can load the car. His eyes get big when he looks at the mounds of stuff I am taking for the party.

"Really? Do you think this is all going to fit in the car?" he asks me. "How are we going to fit any presents she gets?"

I walk over to him and give him a hug, kissing his neck and whispering in his ear.

"I want to do this, please make it fit."

His hand slips down to my bottom and into my back pocket. He pulls me in closer and whispers back to me. "You'll make it up to me later."

"Don't I always?" I say as I kiss him on the lips.

At that moment Adele walks into the kitchen and gives us an "Ewww!" and tells us we look gross and that we're weird too. Richard and I laugh. We kiss again in front of her to irritate her more. She smirks and I tell her it is almost time to go so she should get her coat because we are leaving soon. She excitedly runs upstairs to grab her things.

We arrive early at the youth center for setup and haul in all the baskets of goody bags, cheese puffs, and food. Adele carefully carries in her rainbow colored birthday cake. The supervisor of the youth center tells us she will be back at the end of the party to lock up. We thank her and I quickly begin to hang up balloons, streamers, and more decorations, and then I put the *Grease* soundtrack on the CD player. The upbeat energy is now fully blasting throughout the youth center.

The children arrive as if all at once. I'm not totally ready for the party either. All the little details of putting the games out and making the place perfect aren't finished. However, I have learned only recently that my old self is never finished with completing details. There always is another detail to take care of, and yet another, and then another. My new self actually comes forth during this limboland time of mine and tells me it is okay and to lighten up. There comes this awareness, awakened self, and good-natured feeling about life. I become more lighthearted, playful, and accepting of all things. This is huge, since it has been my number one emotional issue for most of my adult life.

The kids pile their coats on and around the coatrack in a chaotic nine-year-old manner. As each child comes through the door, I notice their faces. Their eyes are big and full of life and they immediately pick up on the liveliness in the air. I notice all the good things, like how one of the cute boys from her school comes over to Adele and touches her shoulder as he wishes her Happy Birthday. I love the way Adele smiles shyly at him and is well-mannered and almost grown-up.

One of her friends, Caitlin, actually hugs Adele and picks her up off the floor. She bends backwards with Adele stiff in her arms. "Happy Birthday, Adele," she screeches. Caitlin shakes Adele's small frame back and forth and then puts her down as they both giggle.

I love every precious moment. They come one after another and I am present with them all day. The party is the perfect nine-year-old birthday celebration. It is better than I could have expected. I treasure that, for the most part, I am not in my head with my thoughts. I don't run with all the "What if's"; I simply enjoy the event.

In the middle of all the kid commotion, and after my duties as birthday mother seem to be taken care of, I ask my husband to dance. While the CD plays "Those Magic Changes" by Sha Na Na, he takes my hand out to one side and I put my other hand around his neck. We continue to dance old fashioned-like and we are in tune with one another as our bodies sway to the old song. I see Adele smile, and while we dance she points at us and grins to her friends. I can tell that she is proud of our family and our togetherness.

As a child, I remember loving to watch my parents dance. My mom and dad would move the kitchen table back so they could polka to the tunes coming out of the old radio, one that had a bent hanger sticking out where the antenna used to be. On Sundays, my mom would fine-tune the AM dial until she found the Polish Polka hour. It came in with white noise but there was no mistaking the accordions. She'd turn it up louder. Lit cigarettes would be on the table in a tin ashtray. There were also a few leftover Old Milwaukee bottles from the night before. It was heavenly, watching them polka. I loved to watch their synchronization flow from the kitchen and into the dining room. My big brother and I would sit with my younger brother and sister, clapping and smiling and waiting for a turn with one of them.

Sometimes Mom and Dad would take all of us kids along to the occasional Polish wedding. When a polka came on—look out! Mom and Dad would dance and twirl, one-two-three, one-two-three, one-two-three. My dad always looked so handsome in his blue suit and his slicked back hair, while Mom would have on her favorite polyester dress with stripes. It twirled perfectly with their harmonized steps.

By the time I was eight years old, I could easily polka with both my mom and dad. We would do our one-two-three step and I would be in fast sync with them. However, whenever I tried to polka with anyone else, like a friend or relative, our coordinated dance usually flopped and fell apart, and we would laugh, attempting to polka again, looking at our feet, and repeating one-two-three, one-two-three, one-two-three.

~ ~ ~

The following Monday, we have Adele's parent-teacher conference at her school. I travel from my school and meet my husband and daughter in the parking lot. Normally, I'd be all wound up before these conferences, ready to trump anything negative the teacher says about my child with my own educational philosophy. But today I'm not wound up. At this point in time, "limboland time," I really don't care about any school's current ELA program or the newest and greatest way to teach math. I decide that I don't care all that much about what my child scored on a test anymore. Mostly, I decide that I want my children to be happy. Perhaps, if a person is happy, this could lower their chances of getting cancer. So I think, *What about that thirteen percent of BRCA1 positive people, the thirteen percent that never actually got cancer?* From where I stand, I assume they're happy people with healthy lifestyles. So my newest and greatest parenting message switches to, "Be happy, love what you do, and be healthy."

Adele's teacher greets the three of us as we arrive. It's a quick conference and her teacher gives us the same message as all the other teachers have given us these past few years: Adele needs to practice her math at home and needs to stop talking during class.

I realize that Adele will never stop talking at school. That's who she is. My kids have always talked incessantly. Ever since they were babies, when they found out they could make a sound with their vocal cords, it's been nonstop. If I were her teacher, I'd have her incessantly explaining math facts to the less academically inclined students. And, as far as practicing math facts at home goes, we'll see. I've made an attempt at the flashcard thing. Maybe I could get Richard to practice math with her or I could get her a tutor. But, having a full-time job, two children at home, dinners that need to be made, gardens that need to be harvested, pets that need to be fed, and bills that need to be paid, seems busy enough. I think that working with the kids on respect and responsibility in the home is a full-time job. Practicing math facts at home is low on my list of priorities.

On the way home from the conference, I ask Adele about who she likes to sit with at lunch and who she likes to play with on the playground. Once we get home, we sing Happy Birthday at our kitchen table and eat homemade cupcakes. In the evening, I tuck Adele into bed. We pray, "God, we pray for our happiness. May we be full of love and health and offer everyone a smile. May we continue to give our best at school, at work, at home, and in this life." Kissing her head I add, "Goodnight my little Poopaa, I love you!"

~ ~ ~

November 10, 2009

The following day I have my cancer tests. I take the afternoon off from work and arrive at the hospital fifteen minutes early. I check in at radiology and I'm first taken to the ultrasound room where they perform a transvaginal ultrasound. I get to keep my upper clothes on but I'm asked to remove everything from the waist down. We make some small talk as I try to figure out what a transvaginal ultrasound is really about. The radiology technician explains that he will be inserting the scope and rolling it over my ovaries to see if there are any concerns. He says this as he holds up a long, thin metal instrument which is attached to a flexible metal hose. On the end of it is a small scope that looks like a roll-on from a perfume bottle. He shows me the latex covering which goes over the scope and then squirts some gel over the instrument.

I lie back nervously and he inserts the scope. I am uncomfortable; who wouldn't be with a tiny camera poking around their ovaries? I notice that he doesn't really watch what he is doing. Rather, he looks at the computer screen that sits next to me, near my head. I try to lift myself up and look at the screen too.

"Do you see anything?" I ask.

"Just normal cysts, nothing abnormal at all."

I immediately like this fellow. He is not a radiologist, and only radiologists read the pictures. However, I can tell he has worked this job a long time and feels comfortable telling people when he sees that things are "normal."

"All done," he says as he finishes taking pictures. He slowly removes the scope and then helps me to sit up. He hands me a thin linen sheet and then a hand towel to clean up all of the extra gel that got on the inside of my thigh. "I'll be back in a minute. You can go ahead and get dressed. I'll walk you to your next test."

We walk together through the large radiology department, first down one hall, then down another. I feel like I'm in a small city in *Star Wars* because people are walking around appearing alien-like, with blue sterile covers on their feet or their heads, or both. I make the parallel thought and realize that in my teaching career, I think kids crying "I want my mommy" and someone walking around in a panther costume is normal too. He gestures me toward a nice young man behind another counter.

"Well, here you are. Jason will take care of you from here. Have a good day."

"Thanks for walking me here," I say with a smile. I don't know if I would have found it myself." I chuckle, trying to remain positive about all of these procedures. I then turn to Jason.

"Your name?" he asks me.

"Angela Fishbaugh."

He puts another hospital band on my wrist and asks, "Your date of birth?"

I tell him. He examines the band and then securely presses the tape to my small wrist.

I joke, "Hey, these are just like the ones from the amusement park."

He half smiles and walks to a room behind the counter and comes back shortly with the smoothie drink. He hands it to me. "This is for the upper MRI. You can drink the other half at three o'clock." He reaches under the counter and pulls out a clipboard. He slides it towards me. "I need you to fill out some papers."

I sit down in the waiting room. There is no one else here. I finish the papers, drink my smoothie, close my eyes, and think, *I have been visiting hospitals my whole life.*

I remember visiting my dad in many different hospitals after he left Willard Psychiatric. He was being sent to other hospitals to check for other medical reasons that might be causing his unusual behavior. Syracuse, New York, was only the second major city I had driven in all by myself, and Syracuse's Upstate Medical Hospital was in itself like its own *Star Wars* city.

When I arrived at the hospital, I closed the ashtray to hide any left-over roaches that Uncle John might have forgotten. I locked the car and put my purse on my shoulder, trying hard to look like a native city girl rather than a country bumpkin. I put on my sunglasses to hide my blood-shot eyes and miraculously ended up on the right floor to visit my dad. He was in a private room all by himself, sitting up, wearing the same tan golf shirt that I had seen him in for years. Unfortunately, he didn't look as buff and young as he used to. Instead he looked weak and pale.

Deep within, I felt something was seriously wrong but I just couldn't put my finger on what it was. I thought perhaps it was the medication they had him on. He was sitting upright, in a straight back chair, and looked incredibly uncomfortable. I wondered why someone who was uncomfortable wouldn't move to get comfortable.

Dad's hair also looked a bit greasy; his grayish-white complexion appeared hungry for the sun, and his overall demeanor seemed starving for life. When I walked into the room he smiled and asked where I had been. I immediately felt guilty for not being there sooner to visit. *Thank God I'm here,* I thought. *Thank God someone is here.*

Why wasn't Dad wondering where the hell everyone else was? Where the hell was Mom and her drugged-up Valium self? I traveled two and a half hours and my nineteen-year-old self was already looking forward to getting back into some lively club scene where lights were flashing, people were dancing, and I could drown this memory of impending doom.

However, my maturity took over. I stayed and talked about whatever came to Dad's mind that day. He shared what he wanted to do when he got out of the hospital. He talked about taking me to Poland to visit where his family came from. It was so depressing. First, because he didn't have a job and had just gotten out of a psychiatric hospital, so there was no way in hell he could take me to Poland. More importantly, the sadness stemmed from my heart because I could already see where this was all heading; not a travel agent or a family reunion, but rather some unknown place that I was deeply afraid of, that my mom was avoiding, and that anyone who was living was afraid to be around.

After hours of visiting, I kissed my dad on the head and helped him get comfortable. He got into the bed and I took off his socks and rubbed his feet. I massaged and massaged and then covered his feet with the white cotton hospital blanket. I then kissed the top of the blanket where his feet were now resting. "I'll be back this weekend," I promised.

"Do you have to go already?"

"I do, Dad."

He smiled and said, "I love you, Poopaa."

I cried as I tried to find my car in the hospital parking lot. After somehow managing to find it and then finding my way out of the parking garage, I checked for highway coins and for the tollbooth card, noticing the roaches in the ashtray. I turned on the radio, which was worth more than the car itself, and tuned it to hear the song more clearly. Journey's "The Wheel in the Sky" was playing. The late August sky looked mystically divine with the sad gray colors mixing with the bright hues of peach and rose. I wiped my tears and couldn't wait to reconnect with my friends. I took a big drink of water and felt spiritually strong after the day's dedicated-daughter time at the hospital. I headed towards home for the two-and-half-hour trip.

I open my eyes when a new man in hospital scrubs comes into the waiting area to take me for my next test. It is time for my three-thirty abdominal/pelvic CAT scan. I get to keep all my clothes on but I need to remove all jewelry and electronic devices. They insert an IV in my arm and before he presses a start button he tells me it is going to feel like I am wetting my pants. He starts the IV and I immediately feel this peeing sensation down below. They tell me to listen to the machine and hold my breath when it instructs me to do so. He adds that I should hold very still and do as the machine says.

Everyone leaves the area. The bed rolls me halfway into a highly sophisticated contraption with a large, circular opening. The machine tells me to breathe, then to hold my breath. I see a circle of red lights, which flash quickly during this procedure. Once the flashing has finished, the machine once again says "breathe," which I do.

Partway through the test, two men behind some glass speak into a room speaker.

"Angela, you doing okay?"

With my hands behind my head and holding as still as I can, I shout back, "I'm okay."

The bed takes me in and out, and we repeat this several times. I hold my breath, pictures are taken, and then I am asked to breathe again. Finally, one of the men behind the glass tells me we're finished. He comes in and takes my IV out as he helps me to sit up.

"Are you doing okay?" he asks me again, and I tell him that I'm fine.

Afterwards, he leads me to where I will have my upper MRI. We walk down the hallway and into a locker area where I can go behind a curtain and remove everything but my underwear. I am again asked to remove my earrings and cell phone and my wedding band too. I feel vulnerable and strong at the same time as I neatly tuck these items into my boots at the bottom of the locker. I walk out wearing a hospital gown and he takes me into the next room where the upper MRI machine is ready for me, along with another woman in scrubs. I look down and and see that there is a narrow padded gurney for me to lie on, face down. This bed is also on rollers and is part of the large MRI machine. There is an area just below the head part that cannot be mistaken for what is supposed to go in it: breasts. My own are so small that I point at the hollowed area and make a joke.

"You think my breasts are going to fit through those holes?"

The nurse's partner smiles. "We've heard it all. Okay Angela, can you tell me your date of birth?"

I turn to her and say, "I hadn't realized this upper MRI is for breasts only. Can it also tell if there are issues regarding your lungs or surrounding area?"

The man answers for her as he points for me to sit on the table. "We can sometimes see a mass if it is around the breast area but this is predominately an MRI for breasts. Are you having lung problems?"

"No," I say before continuing to explain. "But my father died of lung and brain cancer at the age of forty-two and I thought the doctor would have ordered an MRI that looked at everything in my upper body."

The nurse reassures me. "This is a state-of-the-art machine, the best they have, and it will be able to detect if there are any concerns." As he explains this, the woman makes a note in my file regarding my dad's cancer.

I like these two people and feel reassured. They explain that this is about a forty-five minute procedure. I will be lying face down with headphones on and if at anytime I feel scared or uncomfortable, I can squeeze the ball in my hand and a bell will go off to alert them that I need to come out. They make it clear that the MRI is very loud and that is why I will have headphones on. They ask me what kind of music I like and I tell them classic rock. I lie face down with the headphones on and do my best to put my breasts in the holes. The man and the woman, each on either side of me, make some adjustments to my breasts underneath the table. They place the squeeze ball in my hand and ask me, through the speakers in my headphones, if I'm doing okay. They adjust the volume of the classic rock station and roll the gurney and me into the narrow tube. Once inside, I can see my face, cradled in the gurney, reflected on a piece of shiny metal in the bottom of the machine. I'm helplessly strapped in and feel like crying. Instead, I breathe in, close my eyes, and wish they would have had machines like this in 1987.

"The Tide Is High" by Blondie plays in my ears, and I think perhaps my dad wouldn't have died so quickly if he had had a highly sophisticated machine like this during the time of his cancer. The song was one of his favorite pop hits in the eighties. When I was a teenager, in the car with him, he would turn up the radio when it came on. He'd grab my hand and hold it up in the air like a victory celebration and say "Hey, it's the 'I'm going to be your number one' song." I would smile every time and shake my head at him.

"Dad, c'mon, you know it's called 'The Tide Is High.'" It always made me feel wonderful that he wanted to be my number one.

A tear drops to the bottom of machine and lands on the metal mirror. I see the splash and I feel a lump in my throat as I hold back my other tears. I close my eyes tighter and swallow my feelings.

I remember the early fall day in '87 when I found out my dad had cancer. My boyfriend Al and I were sound asleep in a sleeping bag on my living room floor, sprawled out on the thin brown Berber carpet. It was a large room with dark paneling and only had one piece of furniture in the center of it, just the middle piece from a three-piece, 1970s sectional sofa. A tiny ten-inch, black-and-white television sat on top of a wooden box in the corner. It had a bent hanger where the antenna was supposed to be, just like my parents' radio.

When the phone rang early that morning, I noticed that the TV was still on. I realized it had to be very early because only white noise and snow appeared on the screen. I reached over Al and grabbed the rotary phone that had a thirty-foot cord coming from the kitchen.

"Yeah Ang, it's Mom," an angry-sounding voice said when I picked up.

"What's going on, did they find anything out?"

My mom began crying. "Your father has cancer. I don't know what I'm going to do."

My body became numb and I felt my heart begin to pound. I opened my mouth to say something, but nothing came out. I cleared my throat and muttered, "What? Cancer? Where?"

Mom's voice sounded angry again. "They think it's a brain tumor. They are going to do more tests. I just don't need this right now. When can you come back to the hospital?"

As dysfunctional as my family always seemed to be, there was one thing that was absolutely certain: we were always there for one another. If a tragedy arose, we held our heads high and clung together like the Polish clan that we were.

"I'll come right now," I said.

I kissed Al's forehead and told him I had to go to the hospital. He rubbed his eyes and climbed out of the sleeping bag.

"I'll put oil in the car," he said gently.

This continued for the next eight months: Put oil in the Pinto while a cigarette hung out one side of my mouth. Eat fast food while driving. Go see Dad in the city hospital, either by myself, with my brother, my uncle, or both. Calm Mom down or argue with her to stop taking so many pills. Go check on my younger teenage brother and sister when I returned home each evening. Sleep in the sleeping bag with Al. Then, every few days, call in sick to work. Again and again and again.

"Angela, we're done. We're going to pull you out now," the MRI technician's voice suddenly comes through my headphones.

Once I'm out and away from the machine, I sit up, put my arms across my chest, and break out into a sobbing cry.

"Are you okay? What's wrong?"

Weeping, I simply come out with, "I miss my mom and dad."

They hand me a tissue and tell me to take my time. The woman rubs my back and says, "You sure have been through a lot today."

I sure have been through a lot in this life, I think to myself.

I get composed and when I look at the clock I realize I'm done a bit early. I've scheduled to meet two friends at the Elbow Room, a bar next to the hospital. This is my reward. I don't ask anyone to take me to all of these tests but I do have some friends who will gladly meet with me afterwards for a drink near the hospital. Because I am done a little earlier than planned, I walk to the hospital's gift store and buy the last five of their pink rhinestone breast cancer necklaces. I plan on giving them to five of my friends at school. I actually want six, but they only have five, so I also buy a breast cancer bracelet for my other friend.

I meet Pam and Francine at the Elbow Room and we order wings, jalapeño poppers, beer, and some other deep-fried food. We joke with the waiter, "Can you deep fry our beer and the blue cheese too?"

While at the bar, I order another drink and see the man who took care of me during my CAT scan.

"I took care of you today," he shouts when he notices me.

I feel like Angela again, now that I am out of the hospital gown and in my knee-high boots, tights, and knee-length skirt. I hold my beer up to him with gratitude.

"Thanks again."

Francine and Pam are on edge and ask if I know anything yet. I tell them I just had the tests a few hours ago and it's time to drink beer. Francine agrees but returns to the question anyway.

"What is going on?" she asks.

I try my best to explain but I can tell my friends are baffled by BRCA genetic knowledge as they continue to ask the same question several times. "But you don't have cancer right now, correct?"

I repeat the same answer.

"No. However these tests will provide more information in the next few days."

We drink our beers, eat the chicken wings and poppers, and everyone laughs when I casually share, "Listen, none of us are getting out of this life alive."

Afterwards, we walk to the parking lot together. It is a mild evening and the stars are twinkling in the sky. We hug one another and earnestly share, "I love you."

I listen to the classic rock station on the way home and hear the same song playing from during my breast MRI—"The Tide Is High," by Blondie. My dad's favorite song has now been given to me two times on this particular day. I feel this is no coincidence and find it to be quite amazing and auspicious. I am immediately awakened to his spiritual presence again. I smile and raise one hand in the air. I feel a tingle go down my spine and throughout my whole body. "I get your message, Dad! I love you!" I turn up the volume and sing along, "I'm gonna be your number one . . . The tide is high but I'm holdin' on . . ."

6

In My Own Shoes

November 11, 2009
The next day I go to work and do my job well. I notice I'm more present during my limboland time. I laugh with the students and see special moments everywhere I turn. I notice kindness in the kids, and I notice kindness in myself.

My assistant asks me every few hours about my health. I can tell she is trying to piece this one together. She knows I have had an abnormal pap smear and she knows I am being tested for cancer. She seems more giving and routinely tells me to take breaks, saying that she can take care of this or that task at work. The next few days are only filled with kindness in my mind. Of course, the occasional "What if" thoughts came along here and there too.

I meet with Dr. Dayes late in the day so I don't have to take off anymore work. It is a quick 4:00 p.m. appointment and I arrive on time and say hello to both the receptionist and Leigh, who then takes me right back to the patient room. Dr. Dayes follows her immediately after she has taken my vitals.

"All the tests are negative. You don't have cancer," he says happily after flipping through my file.

I'm completely relieved and blow out a long sigh. "Oh thank God."

Dr. Dayes fixes his glasses. "Yes, this is very good, but you are positive for BRCA1." He clears his throat. "It's not a matter of *if* you get cancer, it's now about *when* you will get cancer." He completes his thought by adding, "I'm recommending a mastectomy followed by a TAH/BSO—a hysterectomy."

My smile quickly fades and I try to reason. "So, because Hereditary Breast and Ovarian Cancer syndrome still exists as part of my genetic makeup, you think I should have a mastectomy *and* a hysterectomy?" My mind still cannot wrap around the fact that I need to remove my breasts even when there is no disease in them.

He reminds me again. "It's not about *if* you get cancer, it is about *when*." He raises one finger and points at me, giving me his stern father stance. "Don't wait on this."

Dr. Dayes tells me that he can do the hysterectomy and Leigh can schedule it. He explains how he will go through my abdominal wall during the procedure and that I will need a six week recovery time at a minimum. I ask about alternative ways since I am an avid exerciser and six weeks seems like an eternity to me. That's when he mentions robotic surgery. He seems excited to share his knowledge about this type of surgery, explaining how five small incisions would be made on my abdomen and how the surgeon isn't even in the room during the procedure. Rather, during the surgery, they will be running the robotics from another room. This sounds intriguing to me; I would much rather have five small incisions than one long six-inch gap that will take longer to heal. The robotic surgery sounds quite impressive, highly sophisticated, and futuristic.

I am able to accept the fact that I need a hysterectomy because I've had painful periods since I was thirteen, I am done with childbirth, and because I know several women who are completely satisfied that they underwent a hysterectomy. I know I need to determine what type of procedure to use to complete it, whether it be robotically or the traditional abdominal way. But, when it comes time to discuss the mastectomy part of my decision, I want to sweep that idea under some carpet and pretend it doesn't even exist. When I offhandedly try to ignore the mastectomy part of his recommendation, Dr. Dayes again slowly shakes his finger at me and bluntly says, "Don't let this go, don't let this go. You need to take care of it."

When I got home in the evening, I inform Richard of every detail. I share first and foremost that I am clear of any cancer in my body. Then I explain how Dr. Dayes wants me to have both a mastectomy and a hysterectomy as a preventive measure. Although this isn't the first time Richard has heard me discuss all of this, I can tell it now all feels too much for him.

After being married for nearly twelve years, I can tell when it all just seems like too much for Richard, just by his subtle body language.

He always starts to multitask during critically important moments in the conversation, like fidget with the recyclables under the sink. I'll be talking about having a preventative mastectomy and then he'll just blurt out something inappropriate like, "Boy, these recyclables are overflowing, I better take care of them."

As his wife, who is also a therapist, it is my job to reel him back to reality.

"You know what else is overflowing, our emotions, these important decisions." Then I use Dr. Dayes's words. "It's not about *if* I get cancer, it's about *when* I get cancer."

Richard stops his multitasking and holds out his arms. "Baby, you know I'll support whatever it is you decide."

Once Richard and Adele go to bed, I pour a glass of wine and stay up late researching on the computer: *BRCA1* positive, proactive mastectomies, hysterectomies, healing times of the robotic surgery, the traditional hysterectomy, and the mastectomy operations. Then I come back to *BRCA1* positive research and realize that it doesn't lie. All of the reliable cancer research, every trustworthy internet page I go to, from the American Cancer Society to breastcancer.org, all offer the same alarming statistics: About 5–10 percent of breast cancers can be linked to gene mutations (abnormal changes) inherited from one's mother or father. Mutations of the *BRCA1* and *BRCA2* genes are the most common.[1]

During my research, I pause for a moment. I close my eyes, take in a breath, and reflect on my mother's breast cancer, my father's lung and brain cancer, my grandmother's breast cancer, my other grandmother's uterine cancer, and my uncle's colon cancer. I simultaneously see all of their uphill battles in my mind. I take one last sip of my red wine and feel deep within that I never want an uphill battle. Life is difficult enough at times. I can tolerate downhill battles better—who couldn't? It's a better fight. So I decide on the proactive decisions and shutdown my computer for the evening. I put my wineglass in the sink and head to bed. Tomorrow is Friday, thank God! I have one more day of pre-K and then my hair appointment in the afternoon. I think how nice it will

---

[1] This information was taken from Breastcancer.org and is current as of this book's publication date. More information can be found using the sources listed in the back of the book.

be to talk to one of my oldest friends, Maureen, who has been doing my hair these last twenty years. It's near midnight as I walk upstairs.

~ ~ ~

November 13, 2009

Today is my dad's birthday. He would have been sixty-four years old. Throughout my workday, I remember this fact. After work, I stay in the parking lot in my car and call Leigh at Dr. Daye's office, with whom I am happy to talk. She has been working at setting up dates for me while I've been taking care of the youngsters at school. Leigh has scheduled a December 2 hysterectomy for me and a second opinion regarding the mastectomy recommendation for 1:00 p.m. on Monday, November 2, with a breast specialist in Corning, New York. This means I need to take a half sick day on Monday for this appointment, which is fine; however, it just adds to the stress level since I am a super responsible worker who usually shows up to work even when I am virtually on my deathbed. Leigh also helps me out by providing me with a Rochester phone number so I can get a second opinion from Dr. Murphy, an oncologist OBGYN.

I am beginning to like Leigh more every day as she obviously really cares and wants to help in any way she can. I call Dr. Murphy's office in Rochester to schedule a consultation for the second opinion I want regarding my hysterectomy decision. Basically, I want Dr. Murphy to look at my file and give me the thumbs up for a go ahead with, "Yes, Angela, this is a good decision."

However, there is a setback because, when I call Dr. Murphy's office, the secretary says she can't see me until the end of December. I start to cry.

"What do you mean? I've just scheduled a hysterectomy for early December and I only need another opinion since I've tested positive for BRCA1." I practically beg. "Perhaps Dr. Murphy could call me. We could do a phone consultation?"

The secretary responds coldly. "You don't have cancer and Dr. Murphy gives people who have cancer top priority right now. Nor would Dr. Murphy ever talk cancer issues over the phone." She finishes unemotionally. "I will call you if there are any cancellations."

I give her my cell phone number and end the call in tears. I sit in the parking lot sobbing and questioning all my medical plans.

I suddenly feel my mom and dad in the car with me, and an instantaneous sense of relief comes over me. I take a deep breath and pull myself together by thinking I can take care of part of this on Monday when I go see the breast specialist. It is the weekend and I will begin it by driving to get my haircut.

Every time I go to Maureen's Lakeview Hair Design, I tell my family I am going to my "hairapy" appointment. And therapy it is! Maureen has been cutting my hair since we were thirteen years old. I can't wait to see her. She is one of my oldest, dearest friends and always knows how to make me feel better. I trust her with all my innermost anxieties. I need to tell her everything that is going on in this hectic life of mine, about all these tests I've endured and that I am waiting on. I want to tell her about the cold secretary who wouldn't get me in for an appointment. I like hanging out with Maureen because I get to revert to my teenage self. I can use words like, well, badass teenage words that you wouldn't say around your parents.

I want to also tell her that it is Dad's birthday today and that he has been gone for twenty-one years and that I miss him. She will understand. My dad loved Maureen. He gave her a made-up Polish name since Maureen wasn't typical of Polish. He called her, "Nanewshka," which was eventually shortened to "Newnee."

Maureen's husband, Gary, is also a dear friend. I explain everything to both of them when I arrive for my haircut, leaving nothing out. I go on to tell them about my upcoming colonoscopy, my approaching appointment with the breast specialist, and the woman in Rochester who was so cold to me. They listen and, more importantly, support me.

When I ask Gary what he thinks of all this, he shakes his head as if he can hardly believe it all. "Go for it! I would if I were in your shoes."

"Yeah, we want you around!" Maureen adds.

Before I leave the salon I receive a call from the secretary at Dr. Murphy's office, but this time the secretary sounds warm.

"Angela," she says kindly, "I can get you in Monday at 9:00 a.m."

"This Monday?" I ask hopefully.

"Yes, this Monday, November 16. We had a cancellation."

I'm grateful for the news. "I'm sorry about earlier on the phone, this has been just so much for me," I add wholeheartedly.

She reassures me. "No problem, I'm sorry too. I'm glad I could fit you in. We'll see you on Monday."

When I hang up, I look at Gary and Maureen with amazement,

"I think this appointment was my dad at work!" I look up to the ceiling and with my hands in prayer I thank God. "Happy Birthday, Dad! I love you!"

Maureen and Gary each give me a hug and Maureen tells me she'll call me this weekend. I drive home with Pearl Jam's "Alive" cranked up on the radio.

This period of time, the time where I know I don't have cancer and am about to make major decisions about proactive surgeries, is chock-full of opinions. Everyone I talk with has an opinion to add. I love my family and friends with all my heart but no one in my inner circle has truly ever heard about proactive genetic testing and proactive surgical procedures.

One of my friends has a judgmental look on her face as I try to explain that I'm thinking about having a mastectomy even though I didn't have cancer. She shares that I should get another opinion. A colleague from work says she thinks this is all awesome because I can do something about cancer before cancer even comes. She adds that I should have the operations within the next year. I visit my massage therapist and he almost turns me away because he is not allowed to work on anyone with cancer. I explain that I don't have cancer, rather more than an eighty percent chance of getting it. He reluctantly gives me my massage and afterwards, while writing him a check for the visit, he tells me I should go to the Sloan Kettering Hospital in New York City.

My brothers and sister and cousins listen to my woes as well. My younger brother, Anthony asks, "Do you have to have chemo?" I realize he didn't understand anything I told him. Later I find out, through the family grapevine, that he's told one of his friends when they ran into each other while pumping gas at a gas station, that I have cancer. I call him as soon as I hear this and instruct him not to tell anyone that I have cancer. All this *BRCA1* information seems too futuristic and intense for him. He can't even wrap his mind around the new genetic testing technology. During the phone conversation, he asks if I have to have radiation therapy and I just roll my eyes as I again tell him not to tell anyone I have cancer.

My Aunt Deb tells my Aunt Eva that I should only get the hysterectomy and not the mastectomy. My Aunt Eva then calls me and tells me she agrees with Aunt Deb. Later in the week, my Aunt Eva calls me again and says she talked to her friend who worked at a hospital in Chicago and now she agrees with me and that I should have both surgeries. My husband Richard says people think a hysterectomy is nothing because you can't see internal organs ripped away when you are walking around. But you can see that your breasts have been removed. He advises me to use only my own wise logic, that it is better than anyone else's opinions. He tells me to keep trusting my gut.

On Saturday, I meditate all by myself. Usually I meditate with my husband at five in the morning before work. Monday through Friday, we sit in silent meditation, say a prayer, read an inspirational excerpt in a book from our family library, and finally give each other a morning hug to start off our workday.

This morning, I decide to move my meditation cushion to the middle of the room and position myself so I can view my T-junction road sign painting that symbolizes the need to make a decision. After ten or so minutes of focusing on my breathing, an enlightened thought comes to me: "A mediocre decision made in a timely manner is better than a perfect decision made too late."

I heard this quote a year or so ago when it came up in a phone conversation I was having with my cousin Jim. My cousin had a lifelong career in the Navy; twenty-four dedicated years to be exact. We talked about once a week and usually got entangled in conversations that were quite interesting, whether they were political, about family, about alternative music we liked, or any current affairs in the world. During this particular conversation, Jim was telling me that the manner in which I lived my life—by making decisions and moving forward—was impressive. He told me then that this quote was something Navy men lived by.

Jim always had strength and kind words to share with me. I had not thought of that conversation in a long time, nor had I ever been able to draw up that quote to save my life. But this day, during this quiet day of peaceful morning meditation, it comes to me. Today I firmly decide I will have both preventative surgeries. I make the decision to write them in stone by calling the hospital this week and getting these surgeries on my calendar.

When I walk downstairs, I immediately tell my husband about my meditative experience and my decision to move forward with both surgeries. He supports me and gives me a hug. I pour a cup of coffee for myself and I feel good about my decision.

On Sunday I meditate again. I take off my slippers and set them by my bed. I continue to position myself so I can see the road-sign painting. While I meditate, I feel good and secure about my decision, however I notice some discomfort come up. I am still uncertain about how to deal with my family's and friends' mixed thoughts about my decision. After several minutes of silence and following my breath, I notice my slippers beside my bed. The slippers look as if there is light around them and then I hear that quiet wise voice inside whisper, "No one has to walk in your shoes. Only you have to walk in your shoes." From that moment forward it is easier for me to talk about this life issue with my worried friends and family.

∾ ∾ ∾

November 16, 2009
Monday morning, 5:00 a.m., and I am now sitting in meditation with Richard. My mind mulls over all the questions I will ask the doctors and specialists during today's visit: "Do you think I'm doing the right thing? Would you do the same? If I have my breasts and female organs removed, will the gene want to make cancer somewhere else in my body? What about my kids, my brothers, my sister—should they get tested?"

I am also thinking about the two hour drive to my 9:00 a.m. appointment in Rochester and the following trip back to Corning for my 1:00 p.m. appointment with Vanessa Kerr, the breast specialist. I take a breath and make a mental note in my mind that I should bring extra water and snacks for today's trip. I take another breath and notice gratitude emerging. I feel grateful to have my husband with me at this moment and for our upcoming travel today. Later, when I get my coffee, I give Richard a kiss and tell him this is like a date, a whole day adventure, a medical date.

He hugs me. "I'm sure you'll be taking me on some medical dates in the future," he says.

It has been so ironic that Richard is focusing on my forty-one-year-old health right now. Richard is sixty-five years old and still works very hard. Yes, he is drawing social security, but he's never truly retired. He has always worked for himself as a carpenter's helper and experienced painter. He has done all the remodeling in our beautiful

1830s-era farm home, everything from our hardwood floors to our cabinetry and addition. He thinks nothing of climbing a thirty-foot ladder. He tried using his associate's degree with different traditional jobs around our area but he said that when he worked for others, he always went back to smoking cigarettes very heavily.

He had quit smoking in 1997 when I told him I wouldn't marry him if he smoked. So when we did marry, in 1998, we both agreed that it was more important that he remained healthy and happy in his job, especially since we were twenty-four years apart in age. I loved it that he was in great shape, and I rarely ever thought of the age gap that separated us. However, today is one of those days where the irony of it makes me understand this relationship fact of ours. And since Richard works for himself, he can take off any day he needs. I am so grateful he is with me for these second opinions today.

As we head off in the car, I type Dr. Murphy's address into our GPS. It is a cloudy day, appropriate for my cloudy thoughts. Nothing seems perfectly clear right now. I know I have made the decision to have these proactive surgeries, however I don't know when they will happen and how far apart they will be scheduled from each other. I don't even know who will perform them, and I am not sure about the recovery time either.

I think about how quickly my dad's cancer took him; from diagnosis to death, it was ten months. Ten months consumed with chemo, bloating and sickness, baldness and madness, thinness and sadness, and eventually his death. Twenty-one years later, I can sometimes still feel my head spinning from that family trauma.

My goal today is to get clear and concise answers to my questions. I, of course, never want cancer to take me quickly, leaving my children to process an awful and traumatic event for the rest of their lives, like I have had to. Rather, I am going to act quickly. After all, a critical decision made in a timely manner is better than getting cancer.

We arrive at Dr. Murphy's office where I finally meet the secretary who had initially been so cold to me. She is now extremely friendly and says she is so happy to meet me and that Dr. Murphy will be right out. As Richard and I take a seat, another woman comes into the office with her friend, walks by my seat, and checks in with the secretary. She reeks of menthol cigarettes, just like my mom used to. She coughs and tells the secretary she is here to see Dr. Murphy. Richard is reading a magazine and tries to point out an article about the health benefits of wine. I pretend to be focused on the magazine article while still trying to listen to the conversation the two women are having.

I notice the coughing lady adjust her body, appearing to be extremely uncomfortable in the wooden chairs.

"Dr. Murphy said they got all the cancer," she says to her friend, "but I think it's back. My blood levels were off again." She squirms a little more in the chair and fidgets with her tight fitting jeans, which could be partly the reason for her apparent discomfort.

"Do you want me to go in with you?" her friend asks in a consoling voice.

"Yeah," she says, looking relieved. "And thanks for sticking by me."

Richard points to the article and smiles. "See, wine is good for you. It's good for you, baby!"

"I want you to go in with me today to all of these appointments. I want you to go in with me with everything, okay?" I say to him, ignoring his comment.

"Is that okay to do?" he asks me.

"It doesn't matter if it is okay or not; I just need you to do it."

"Okay, I'll do whatever you want me to do," he says as he taps my arm with his hand. I lean in and rest on his shoulder.

My mom used to cross these types of boundaries all the time, going where she wasn't supposed to go, pushing through to where she wasn't invited. Since I was little, she'd barge in the bathroom when I was taking a bath. The one thing we didn't have growing up was privacy. I thought things would change when I grew up and had my own kids and home, but nope!

I remember one particular night when Mom walked in the house with a lit cigarette in her mouth.

"Where's Ang?" she asked Richard, without hesitation.

Richard, knowing my mom, simply pointed to the stairs and said, "Taking a bath."

So up the stairs she marched, right into my bathroom. I didn't flinch or bother to move anymore. That day, I was soaking in frothy bubbles. I had cucumbers on my eyes, a mud mask on my face, a plastic bag on my conditioning hair, and lemon ice water to sip on.

The moment she barged in, I peacefully said, without removing the cucumbers, "Cigarette, Mom! Cigarette! Please!"

She tossed it in the toilet in her usual aggravated manner. "Oh, Jesus Christ. There, you happy?!"

"What's going on?" I asked nonchalantly, not having moved from my bath.

"I'm not feeling well, Ang."

"For the umpteenth time, just quit smoking," I responded, annoyed.

"Stop, that's not it. I just know my body and feel like something is wrong."

"Well then maybe you need to quit smoking and drinking," I continued.

She closed the toilet cover and sat on top of it, putting her elbows on her knees and resting her chin in her hands. "I just feel like something is wrong."

My mom was a hypochondriac, so I rarely took things that she blurted out seriously. This wasn't always the case, however. When I was seven years old, she shared with me that she was dying from some degenerative disc disease. She told me this while I was petting my kitten and, well, trying to be seven years old. She frantically said this while looking for more pills in her purse. At first I felt very scared and worried that she was going to die the following day. But then later that day, while playing outside, I talked with my brother Ben about it. Ben, who was eleven at the time, explained that Mom was always talking about dying and that I should just plan on it happening for the remainder of my life. So I did.

In the bathroom, I took the cucumbers off my eyes and asked her to hand me a towel. I wrapped the towel around myself as I got out and began to comb my hair.

"I found a lump on my breast," she suddenly said.

She now had my attention. "What? Where?"

She placed her hand over the left side of her fleece sweatshirt. "On this side."

"When did you find it?" I asked.

"Today."

I told her she needed to make an appointment for the following day and get it checked out. She agreed with me, which was unusual. When she left I spanked her on her ass and added, "Quit smoking! At least while you're in this home!" She made a kissing face at me, put a cigarette in her mouth, and winked at me. She told me she'd call me.

A nurse comes out of Dr. Murphy's examination area.

"Angela, Dr. Murphy will see you now."

As I stand up, I motion Richard with my head to follow me. He stands reluctant, not wanting to do anything out of the ordinary or break any boundaries that shouldn't be broken. I check with the nurse to make him feel better.

"I'd like my husband to come with me."

"Absolutely!" she says graciously. "Right this way."

Richard is now at ease as the nurse takes us into a warm, yellow examination room. She asks me a few questions about medications and takes my height and weight. I'm surprised when she doesn't ask me to get undressed or to get into a hospital gown. Instead, she simply says that Dr. Murphy will be with us shortly and then quickly exits the room.

Dr. Murphy enters the room soon after with a clipboard. She is a woman in her fifties, with mousy brown hair, dressed simply, and exuding confidence and light. I feel wonderful in her presence and already taken care of. She shakes my hand, then my husband's, and begins with a well-mannered "I'm glad to meet you. Tell me why you're here today." I run down my August to November saga in as brief a manner as I can, of how my doctor recommended that I have a hysterectomy and a mastectomy. I explain that I am here for a second opinion and then come out with my question.

"Should I get a proactive hysterectomy?"

Dr. Murphy, who has been sitting through my story with her elbows on her clipboard and a smile on her face, suddenly sits upright, takes a deep breath, and asks me a surprising, yet interesting, question.

"Tell me, how is it you came to be tested?"

I tell her all about Dr. Daye's nurse, explain my family's history, and how the nurse thought getting genetically tested would be a good idea in light of my abnormal pap smear.

"Do people not get tested that often?" I ask her.

She tells me that usually people who already have cancer are the ones that get tested. She then clearly explains to me about *BRCA1* and *BRCA2*, using her hands as she talks.

"Out of all cancer patients, only about ten percent are BRCA1 or 2. Once a tumor forms, it begins to grow. We used to think we should only remove the ovaries. However, then we found that in BRCA patients, the tumors began to grow in the fallopian tubes that were left behind after the ovaries were removed. So, later it was decided it was best to remove the ovaries *and* fallopian tubes. However, it was *then* found that BRCA patients developed tumors in their uterus because portions of the fallopian tubes remained there, even after their removal."

She continues to use her hands in a tai chi fashion as she talks more about ovaries, fallopian tubes, uteruses, and the cervix.

"So it was then recommended to have the uterus and cervix removed as well, a TAH/BSO: Total Abdominal Hysterectomy with a Bilateral Salpingo-Oophorectomy."

"So I'm doing the right thing?" I ask as soon as she finishes.

She never says the word yes or points at me like Dr. Daye's has done. Her yes is given by her body language and by her nod. "We know a lot about BRCA1 and 2. We know that this is what happens."

When I ask her about hormone therapy, her expression changes to one of disgust and I immediately understand why. Her face then changes back to the natural tai chi, holistic doctor when she discusses natural supplements, such as extra calcium, vitamin D, and vitamin E. She softens even more as she explains that I will need to take these things instead of hormones. She actually says she despises hormones, especially for BRCA positive patients. So, hormones are out of the question.

"Dr. Dayes told me I could have a 'robotic' surgery. What are your thoughts on robotic surgery?"

She nods. "Yes, I can do a robotic surgery." She explains, by holding up her hand and making about an inch gap between her thumb and forefinger, "There will be five small incisions about this size. They will be in your abdomen and they will be there forever."

"Yeah, but Dr. Dayes said the scars are hardly noticeable."

She nods her head in agreement but wants me to understand clearly. "Yes, they are small, but you will definitely have scars and you will have them the rest of your life."

Dr. Dayes had made it seem like the scars would be unnoticeable. I still lean more towards the robotic surgery though; after all, it's one of only two options being offered to me. I ask her when I can get on the docket to have this all done. She tells me she will walk with me when we are leaving and make sure the nurse looks into it.

Richard and I shake her hand and thank her immensely for her time. We also share that we are on our way to a second appointment today, a breast specialist in Corning, New York. We leave Dr. Murphy's office after booking a January 25 robotic hysterectomy at Highland Hospital in Rochester.

Richard and I discuss how much we like Dr. Murphy during the entire drive down Route 390 to Corning. We arrive an hour and half early, so we stop at the Brewing Company where I order a Blue Moon and a veggie wrap with fries. Richard is eating his tuna melt when he asks, "Do you like how all of this is coming together?"

I take a sip of my beer. "Yes, but I'm going to have to cancel my December 2 hysterectomy at Schuyler Hospital with Dr. Dayes. I don't think he'll mind; he was actually recommending Dr. Murphy and this robotic-type surgery." I take another sip. "Isn't it amazing how doctors can perform robotic surgery? I am so grateful to be alive during this era where so much is possible in the medical field."

"I know! Me too! Just think of my age!" He raises his coffee up to toast with me. "Here's to a good long life together, baby."

The waitress comes over and asks if there is anything else she can get us, before handing us our bill. I shake my head no. "We are wonderful!" I say.

We arrive at Vanessa Kerr's office on time which, we realize, is in the same building as our close friend's physical therapy practice. I sit on the procedure table with my legs crisscrossed and without my shoes on. I am feeling quite relaxed, especially after my Blue Moon. When Vanessa enters, I see she's wearing a long white coat. She has long dark hair and appears to be ten or twelve years older than me. She has a natural elegance about her and I know from Dr. Dayes that she used to work with him but later became a nurse practitioner. She shakes Richard's hand and we make small talk about Dr. Dayes. Then Vanessa asks me, just as Dr. Murphy did earlier, "How did you get genetically tested?"

I explain again how Leigh, from Dr. Dayes's office, offered the genetic test to me. Vanessa, just like Dr. Murphy, reels off information on *BRCA1* and *BRCA2* patients. She explains how it is necessary to stop estrogen in my body as it is a group of hormones in the body that carries information to other cells. It travels in the bloodstream and binds to estrogen receptors. In *BRCA1* positive patients, because there is already a mutation and cells can at some point not be repaired normally, like in typical people, tumors can invasively grow. Therefore, for BRCA positive patients, it is necessary to stop estrogen and not take any forms of it. There will be no hormone replacement therapy for me.

Later I read some articles online that hormone replacement therapy is now okay for BRCA positive patients. However, I take that information just as I take in the vintage newspaper advertisements from the 1940s stating that smoking is good for you. Those old ads conveyed that you could tell if the cigarette was good from your "T" zone, the "taste" and "throat" test. The advertisement has a doctor in a white doctor's coat holding a cigarette up in his hand as he smiles. I clear my throat and firmly make the decision that I will not do hormone replacement therapy either.

"Do you think I'm doing the right thing?" I ask, as I did with Dr. Murphy.

She takes the same stance of not answering directly but nods a firm yes. "We know a lot about BRCA1 and BRCA2. There's even more evidence today that shows its connection with melanoma cancers."

I uncross my legs and sit upright. Looking right at Vanessa I firmly say, "Having a proactive mastectomy can't happen quickly enough for me."

She appears surprised and pleased by my determined response. "Okay then."

"I want to schedule this right away,"

She leaves the room and comes back with a business card. She hands it to me. "This doctor in Pennsylvania can see you tomorrow. You're really going like Dr. Gioe. He's an amazing surgeon."

On our way out of the building we run into our friend, the physical therapist. Richard and I give her the details of why we were in the building today. Before we leave for the day, she also offers her opinion.

"Well, Vanessa is just a nurse. Have you met with a doctor?"

I'm so exhausted that I simply share with her that we were meeting with a third doctor tomorrow to get yet another opinion. Right now, all I want is to get home and make a nice dinner for the family.

On the way home, I call Erica, our secretary at my school, and tell her I need the day off tomorrow as well. I can tell she is concerned. "Angela, is everything okay?"

I tell her that I am going through a lot right now and promise everything will be made clear really soon. I explain that I am not in a position to share everything, at least not yet, and end by telling her that I appreciate all of her help. When I hang up I breathe a sigh of relief. It has been a long day. We've traveled from Dundee to Rochester, to Corning and back to Dundee. I am ready for my living room and my recliner and a glass of Cabernet Sauvignon. I need to sit and relax and feel good about the upcoming plans I am making.

My dad found out he had cancer when it was too far along to actually do anything about it. I can't even imagine what it feels like to be told you have cancer and there is nothing more that can be done. I can't imagine what it feels like to be told it is inoperable and know the disease continues to metastasize throughout your body. I especially can't imagine having a spouse, four children, and a brother living in my home and then being told I'm going to die and wonder how my family will survive without me. How the hell do you plan for that? Dad never had time to make plans or arrangements, to make decisions this way or that. Rather, from the moment he found out, it was an uphill battle. The disease killed him and burned a trauma into the family's heart.

Throughout this, my mother was working two extra jobs. Her regular job as a Certified Nurse's Aide (CNA) was at one of the local nursing homes. She then took on a second job with a home healthcare agency, making minimum wage as a CNA. She drove to people's homes in the evening, feeding, bathing, and putting to bed the handful of elderly people she visited. When she wasn't working, she was sleeping or drinking Old Milwaukee. She had to keep the home running, the bills paid, and food on the table.

My mom also applied for public assistance, which my father despised. He never liked it if anyone couldn't carry their weight, especially financially. He wanted everyone to be self-sufficient. More importantly, he himself wanted to be self-sufficient, and if that couldn't happen, he wanted us to be. At some point, Mom lied to him just so he'd feel better, telling him that we weren't receiving public assistance anymore. Mom didn't qualify for food stamps or heating bill assistance, but the family did qualify for medical aid, which was a huge help during this difficult time.

This time was crazier than any Willard Psychiatric Center days. I lived down the street and was only twenty years old, but I'd taken on the serious role of "immediate health manager" for the Schmidt home. When I entered my family's home, my dad would be lying in his adjustable hospital bed in the living room. He was hairless and the small hospital drawstring pants hung loosely from his body. Woobie, our Chihuahua, was always curled up next to his side. A small table sat beside the bed with his ice water.

On one particular day, Mom was in the bathroom putting on her heavy makeup, getting ready for one of her three jobs. A cigarette hung from the side of her lip while she teased her hair with the white comb. She used an aerosol hairspray and sprayed her entire head while still keeping the cigarette in her mouth. I coughed as I entered the bathroom.

"Jesus, Mom, you're going to blow up the joint. What's going on tonight?"

She was angry already, I could tell by her tone. "Work, just work! Why don't you stick around and see if you can get your dad to eat something, there's applesauce in the fridge. Oh, and check on your sister. She wasn't home last night when I came back from work. She had some story."

I took a drag from my mother's cigarette, "Yuck, menthol," and blew out the smoke. "Okay, don't worry."

I walked out the back door to see where everyone else was. My uncle was on the back porch drinking Old Milwaukee already, while my younger brother was throwing baseballs in the backyard. Now, I know that at first this doesn't sound crazy, but Uncle John was working on a twelve pack of beer, and it was only 11 a.m. And my brother Anthony was throwing baseballs without anyone to catch for him. My dad couldn't play, and, well, Uncle John was "busy." So, my brother threw the baseball at the old shed that sat in the corner of our yard. It used to be a doghouse when our other dog, Peaches, was alive. But Anthony wasn't just throwing the ball; he was pitching it as fast and as hard as he could, smashing it into the old shed. There were already several holes through its wood siding. Then he'd walk to get the ball, go back to his pitching stance, and throw it again. He looked robotic as he did this. Again and again he whipped the ball, like he was working through some internal misery.

This would become the scene, day after day. His anger at his life situation was visibly deforming the shed, eventually leaving the front part of the building looking like the aftermath of the Texas chainsaw massacre. I actually thought that, in some weird way, this was therapeutic for him. So, as the family's "immediate health manager," I never told him to stop.

After checking on the backyard craziness, and after getting a grunt of a response from my uncle, I walked upstairs to see what was going on with my sister. My sister was only fourteen yet was also now smoking. When I walked upstairs, she tried to hide her cigarette by putting the butt in an almost empty Old Milwaukee bottle.

"You better hope Dad doesn't see that," I said to her.

She almost sounded logical when she looked up at me and said, "He can't even make it up the stairs anymore . . . and Mom could give a shit."

I sighed. "Jesus, we got to keep helping each other through this. We got to try."

"Yeah, I know," Chrissy said as she looked down at the floor.

I rubbed her shoulder and told her that I loved her.

I went back downstairs and into the bathroom where Mom was adding more heavy eyeliner.

"Can you just see if he'll eat for you?" she said with a cough.

I nodded and then went to grab some applesauce from the fridge. I sat on the edge of the bed and shooed Woobie to the floor. I rubbed my dad's forehead and brought my hand up over his hairless head.

"Hey Dad, how you doing?" I tried to be cheerful as I scooped up a spoonful of applesauce.

"Pretty good! How are you doing, Poopaa?"

I made small talk with him. "I don't like my job. I wish I had a new one."

He took a small bite of the applesauce. "Don't ever quit one job unless you have another one lined up."

I smiled and scooped up more applesauce for him. "Good advice. Here take another bite." Then I told him about the family. "Anthony is throwing a baseball out back. Boy, he is getting quite the athletic arm."

"How about Chrissy?"

"She's upstairs, acting like a teenager."

Dad took another bite of applesauce. "Poopaa, help them in any way you can. Okay?"

I just smiled at him and nodded yes.

"Where's your mother?"

"Oh, she's getting ready for work." I scooped up more applesauce.

He held his hand up, not wanting anymore applesauce. He looked at me with pain in his eyes. "I wish she didn't have to work so hard," he said.

"I know." I held the straw up to his mouth and gave him a sip of his ice water. Uncle John came into the living room and sat down in the comfy chair next to his bed. I kissed Dad's forehead. "Dad, I'll see you tomorrow. I love you."

He closed his eyes, looked drowsy, and whispered, "I love you, Poopaa!"

John and I gave each other the peace sign, then I patted him on his shoulder as if to say, "Thanks for holding the fort this evening, the kids need you, Dad needs you, and Mom needs you, so don't let your Vietnam vet addictions get to you."

I, like everyone else, knew that Uncle John couldn't stay sober for long periods of time. I liked to believe that because Dad was dying and my younger brother and sister were only fourteen and fifteen years old and my mom was sleepwalking through three jobs, maybe I could trust Uncle John for this brief time of need. I wanted to trust that he could be somewhat mature and trustworthy while my mom went to work. I really wanted to act like a nineteen-year-old and go about my nineteen-year-old life. I had an apartment to look cool in, a boyfriend to hang with. However, I was the "immediate health manager" of the Schmidt family, a role that included a lot of serious responsibilities. Our family home needed so much help and I took on a lot of its responsibility; they needed someone to depend on.

When I left for the evening, I told my sister not to smoke, my brother to be nice to the shed, and my uncle to help everyone out. My mom was leaving too. I slapped her ass as she headed out the door for work. The spank meant "I love you" but was also a reminder about her poor prioritizing regarding this whole situation.

Mom was in denial that Dad was dying; she was in denial that Chrissy was smoking; she was in denial that Anthony was angry and traumatized; and that Uncle John was really not helping with anything since he was smoking pot and drinking heavily. Mom was walking around in a cloud of Valium and Old Milwaukee, purposefully preoc-cupying herself with her work. I wished she could notice the depth of what was going on.

I have somehow always been able to focus on what is going on. Since I was a little girl, I held the major responsibilities in the family. At only six years old, I made everyone's beds. I washed the dishes, made the lunches, did the laundry, dusted, vacuumed, counseled my mom, took care of my younger brother and sister, and barely cried. I barely cried because I was not allowed to. If I cried, Mom usually used this as an opportunity to raise her hand at me and say, "Don't cry or I'll give you something to cry about."

So as a child I was "Super Angie," Mom's "little angel from heaven" who took care of basically everything around the home. I would carry my super responsible disposition with me into adulthood, and into my career teaching little ones to be respectful and responsible.

When it came time to make a decision about Angela, my breasts, my female organs, and planning the itinerary with all these events, it became another serious issue to simply take "super charge" of. I knew how to roll up my sleeves and take responsibility for my life: researching *BRCA1* genes, investigating possible surveillance options, examining different types of surgeries, seeking out all the doctors, making all the appointments, delving into all the necessary questions, studying possible side effects of surgery and medication, and following through to make this all take place was definitely something I could do.

～ ～ ～

November 17, 2009
I meet Dr. Tony Gioe today and it's a day I surely will never forget. I drive myself to the hospital because I need Richard to be at home after work to help out with Adele. Dr. Gioe's office is on the fourth floor of the hospital, and the secretary has me fill out more paperwork again and then check in. When they are ready for me, a nurse comes and gets me from the waiting room. She walks with me down a hallway to a small examination room. I sit there alone and read a breast cancer poster in the office. I always knew there were four stages: stage 1, 2, 3, and 4. However, I didn't know there was a stage 0. I figured my mom was probably late stage 2 or 3 when they found her cancer. I figured this to be true since her cancer had spread to the lymph nodes under her arm.

Dr. Gioe enters the room dressed in jeans and a pair of leather slipper moccasins. He shuffles in with his most sexy, masculine demeanor that hardly can fit through the door. He has on a shirt that is only buttoned up to just over the middle of his chest. He looks like Robert Plant. His hairy gray chest appears ready for some yachting in the Mediterranean. I can tell he likes me immediately by the way he shakes my hand with both of his. His Italian demeanor keeps a light shake going.

"So tell me why you're here today."

I explain everything to him. He seems very intrigued by my story, and in the middle of one of my sentences he stands up and says he'll be right back. Within a few minutes I can hear him outside the door with a few other people. I hear papers shuffling from the clip-board as Dr. Gioe speaks. "We have a BRCA1 positive that doesn't have cancer."

He comes back in the room, this time with a young man in a blue surgeon outfit. Dr. Gioe introduces us, saying that this is one of his top interns. He asks me if he can sit in on this visit today. I agree that it is fine. I realize I am getting special attention because not only am I *BRCA1* positive, but I don't have cancer. This has officially hit me, just how rare *BRCA1* without actually having cancer truly is.

Dr. Gioe is surprised by the fact that I don't yet have cancer and asks how it was that I came to be tested. I again tell the story as if I were telling it for the very first time. He then calls in his nurse and asks her to get someone from Dr. Dayes's office to fax these results to him immediately. I find it interesting that he wants verification that my story is indeed true.

Once everything is verified, I appreciate what he says next. He casually puts his foot up on his knee, leans back with hands behind his head, and says, "You're doing the right thing." I appreciate this mostly because I didn't ask him anything; he just spontaneously offered his opinion.

Thank God! I think. Finally, a doctor who can actually say this without feeling like they're stepping over some boundary.

He explains all of his BRCA knowledge and how he performs about thirty mastectomies a year now. On and on he goes, confirming everything I need to know. However, at the end, a little twist happens. That little twist makes virtually everything fall into place. When I explain that I am planning on having a hysterectomy using robotic surgery with Dr. Murphy in Rochester, New York, he asks, "Why not just have a regular hysterectomy?"

I ask, "You mean abdominally?"

He tosses his hands up like I should already know all this medical jargon. "No, vaginally!"

I'm shocked that no one has ever offered this to me. "I didn't know that I could have a vaginal hysterectomy!" Then I ask, "Do they have to cut me down there, or do an episiotomy, like when I was giving birth?" The questions are now flooding my mind and I come out with all of them as if in one breath: "How do they get your whole uterus, cervix, and ovaries out through your vagina? Wouldn't they have to make a small surgical incision just below the vaginal opening? How the heck do they get all those organs out?"

He seems irritated that this conventional method was never mentioned to me by the other doctors. "Listen, all these new surgeries—including robotic surgery—are hip and new, and when things are hip and new, the doctors want to do these fancy types of surgeries for everything." He talks like my ethnic family, throwing his hands up, tossing them to the side when he doesn't approve of something. He adds, "It is best to do surgeries that work best for patients. Look into having a vaginal hysterectomy. It is a perfectly fine, traditional method, especially when the patient is in good health." He points at me. "And you're in good health!"

Dr. Gioe thinks aloud some more. He questions that perhaps the doctors thought my *BRCA1* results were only of concern rather than absolutely conclusive. Maybe the doctors figured it would be best to do it robotically or abdominally under the assumption that they would be able to see things better using these types of surgeries. Dr. Gioe explains that vaginal hysterectomies have faster recovery times than going through the abdominal wall. He describes how the doctors remove all the female organs by going up through the vagina. Again thinking aloud, he wonders why the doctors wouldn't have recommended this for me in the first place. Then he tosses his hands up again as he says, "If you don't have cancer, there's no reason to not have it done vaginally. If you can have a vaginal hysterectomy, then why not? The less scars, the better."

He sells me on everything he says. So I ask: "This is all great news! Can you do my hysterectomy as well?"

He smiles at me. "I only perform mastectomies."

"Okay, I have one last question then. How long do I need to wait after my mastectomy before I can actually have a hysterectomy?" I'm now shuffling through my purse to find my diary to write this all down. I stop when he pats me on my knee.

"You should give yourself at least eight weeks of recovery time." He pauses to make sure I heard him.

I feel completely comfortable with Dr. Gioe and decide then and there that I want him to do my mastectomy. He explains that he will be working in the operating room with a plastic surgeon and that his breast health navigator, Carol, will set up an appointment so that I can meet Dr. Panilio before I leave Robert Packer Hospital.

Carol comes in and takes all of Dr. Gioe's information. She leaves and returns shortly with a date for my surgery: December 3, 2009, at seven thirty in the morning. Carol tells me that I should head directly to plastic surgery; Dr. Panilio can meet with me right now, in between his other appointments. She walks me out and points which way I should head down the hallway.

When I arrive at the plastic surgery department, I notice a shame come up inside of me. It comes from deep within, just as any shame would. Throughout my years of getting my therapy certification, I have done a tremendous amount of work on my own issues. Shame is a hot topic in therapy world. I had over 450 hours of psychodrama training when I became a Certified Experiential Therapist. Psycho-drama is action-based therapy where clients use spontaneity, drama, and theatre to gain insight into their personal lives. I had so many hours of training that I thought I had put any shame issues to rest. But no, they have only been diminished down to some tiny fragment, ready to be looked at when needed. Today, that miniscule piece of shame, which had lain dormant within my soul, has resurfaced as I check in at the front counter.

I'm not sure what part of my life this fragmented shame was originally attached to. Figuring what part really doesn't matter though. I know that if I try to figure out where the shame came from, then I will just be heading into my head; I will be thinking, analyzing, and avoiding the shame versus working through it.

The most important realization is that shame has been stirred up. I recognize it immediately because I do not want anyone to know that I am in a plastic surgery department. I look around to see if I know anyone in the waiting room even though I am nearly three hours from home. It feels shameful and vain to be here. Visiting Dr. Gioe felt acceptable with my soul and I stamp some approval on that, as if to say, "It is okay to have breasts removed and scars created." But checking in at plastics has a different stamp, one that seems to say, "It is vain to have recon-structive surgery when people around the world are starving."

So shame comes up. My healthy mind starts arguing with it and its toxic attitude. My higher self takes over quickly. "This plastic surgery is good for you, Angela. You're putting a surgical itinerary together to save your life and it includes cutting off your breasts. It's okay to visit plastic surgery. The people here will help you to feel better about your body image after you have made this critical decision about your breasts. You are forty-one years old and you are in the prime of your life. Feeling good is necessary for a healthy life. It's okay to be here."

Thank God for therapy. I love it that shame has little time with me at this point in my decision making. I continue with my process. When the nurse comes to the waiting area and calls my name, I stand up, hold my head high, and don't give shame any more attention, putting it back to sleep again.

I enter the office alone to discuss the importance of reconstructive surgery and how it will help me in my healing process. I have always heard all about the benefits of plastic surgery and how it has helped to improve sexuality and self-esteem in women. In regards to my breasts being removed, I'm not truly worried about the sexuality part. My husband has been very open and honest with me. He's shared that no matter what, we will find ways to fumble through sex without breasts and make each other happy. And truly, the mind is the organ that is the biggest player when it comes to sex. Self-esteem isn't a huge issue for me either. I feel very feminine with my small 36B breasts and I know I don't really need them to feel like a woman.

Dr. Panilio comes in the small examination room where I am waiting. He is of Filipino heritage, is in good shape, and has big biceps. I like him right away, mostly because he makes time for me in his busy schedule. He spends time thoroughly explaining how everything will happen.

He will be assisting Dr. Gioe during the operation. He clarifies that, after Dr. Gioe completes my mastectomy, he will immediately insert tissue extenders where my breasts once were. He explains that tissue extenders are temporary and are hard-shelled, not soft and supple like breast tissue or the implants. They each have a magnetic valve through which he will insert saline in order to extend the tissue over time. Reconstruction takes time. I had originally thought I would have a mastectomy and wake up with brand new pretty breasts. But nope! That isn't how it works.

"The tissue extenders can remain for up to a year," Dr. Panilio explains.

"A year?" I'm surprised anyone would want a hard-shelled object in their body for a whole year and I want to put myself on a time frame. "What is the shortest time I have to keep them in? I really want to have all surgeries behind me as quick as possible." I'm thinking to myself that I don't have a lot of sick time accumulated at work, so I want to use as little as possible. Also, I want to get all this surgery trouble over with and back to my life of writing, artwork, family time, and taking my life for granted. I want all of these operations to be snip, snap, done.

"We can keep the tissue extenders in for as little as eight weeks."

I sigh. "Oh good! I can deal with eight weeks."

"Over the eight weeks, your chest will grow and grow until you like the size of your chest." Dr. Panilio also talks with his hands, swirling his right hand in an ongoing circle as he adds, "Once you are happy with your chest size, you will have another surgery where I remove the tissue extenders and insert the saline implants."

During our conversation, Dr. Panilio has tried to also promote silicone implants but I have heard too many stories of silicone implants going bad, so I opt for saline implants instead.

When I ask him about a new nipple, he shares that he can keep the nipple by having Dr. Gioe do a "nipple-sparing" mastectomy. In this procedure, he would surgically remove all the breast tissue by going through the center of the nipple while still keeping the nipple, something Dr. Gioe hadn't mentioned. Dr Panilio then shares that some breast tissue remains when you keep your own nipple and that there is a very slight chance that cancer could come.

I shake my head no to this option, even though I can tell that Dr. Panilio likes the nipple-sparing operation. I'm sure that he can make my implants look completely natural and perfect, but I immediately make the decision to not keep my nipple. I haven't come this far to lower the chances of cancer to "only a little bit," after all. I am basing my decision on diminishing cancer to the smallest possible chance. If that means not having my own nipple, then so be it.

Dr. Panilio then explains other ways to make a new nipple. He has me stand up and pulls down my pants. He grabs any fat he can from around my belly area and pinches me here and there, explaining how a surgeon usually would be able to do a tummy tuck and take the tissue from there to do the reconstructed breasts. I hadn't realized they could make breasts from the fat in your belly area. But he says there isn't enough body fat there. I just smile.

He reaches over to my groin area and tells me to sit down. He takes his fingers to the skin in my bikini line, the part where my thigh and groin meet. He shows me the loose skin there. He says he can make a nipple from this area. He shows me how it is darker there, just like the nipple I already have. He says it is better than any medical nipple tattoo they can do. The skin can be used as a graft and flap reconstruction. He explains he will make it protrude and that is how it will stay, protruded. I button up my pants and we talk more about all these options.

At this point, the most important part of plastic surgery for me is the potential healing process it will provide. I know I will be grieving the loss of a part of me; my breasts have nursed my children and given them nourishment during my early mothering years. And, as little as my breasts are, and as mismatched as they naturally appear, they are still mine, a part of me. Soon, they will be severed from me and sent to pathology. Plastic surgery seems like the best place to start my transformation back into the healthy woman I want to be. It is a place that can help me to physically be put back together again while I work through the emotional and spiritual aspects of these critical decisions.

That night I go home and look through a book entitled *Show Me*. It is a book of women who have had mastectomies and provides the reader with short stories regarding the patient's cancer, along with visual pictures depicting the whole event, from before, to the surgery, and to after. I am grateful I don't have cancer, because cancer makes a surgeon's job more difficult when they have to work around tumors. I look at all the women's scars and realize Dr. Gioe has given me a gift. If I can have a vaginal hysterectomy I will only have the scars from my mastectomy.

The next morning, I call Dr. Daye's office and make an appointment. He gives me a local surgeon's number who performs vaginal hysterectomies. I think he seems a little disappointed that I'm not having the hip new robotic surgery with the Rochester surgeon. However, when I explain that my decision has to do with wanting less scars, he seems to understand. My decisions regarding my mastectomy and hysterectomy are made.

7

"Inspired"

I've been keeping my boss, Joe, up-to-date with my doctor visits. I think this is necessary since I have been missing so much work for all my appointments. Now that I have truly made all my decisions—that I will be having a mastectomy on December 3, 2009, followed by a hysterectomy on February 3, 2010, along with reconstructive surgery in the third week of February—I fill my boss in during a private meeting. It's the Friday before Thanksgiving and I break down crying as I share everything with him and how all this has been so much on me. I let him know that I will be telling my colleagues next week and he says he wants to be there for me, supporting me as I explain everything to my friends and colleagues.

After our meeting, Joe hugs me and shares that he will keep me in his prayers. I tell him I will send him and the superintendent a letter with all the details. I stay after school and compose everything I know to date. It reads:

Dear Lynn and Joe,

I will need to take two medical leaves this year. The first one will be in December. On December 3rd, I will be having my first major surgery. I plan to call Joe over Christmas break to share how I am feeling and give him a definite date for my return. I am hoping for an early January return (I know the children's lively energy will be a wonderful pick-me-up). My second major surgery, as of right now, is planned for February. However, I will give you more information as it comes in.

Lynn, I have been keeping Joe informed of my health issues; please feel free to get any details from him or me. I'm still processing it all, so it helps me to talk about it as well. I would be happy to talk with you personally too. As a side note, Joe will be supporting me on Monday when I let a small group of my colleagues know more of the "particulars." Joe shared he will be sending a brief note to my families regarding a "generic" medical leave and who will be their child's substitute teacher for this short time.

Another side note, I have thoroughly appreciated Joe's compassion and support these past few weeks. It has made a huge difference in coping with this alarming and recent issue in my life. Thank you Joe, *as always*, for your amazing support.

I appreciate my CSCS family more than you know. I feel very blessed to be a part of this wonderful group for these past thirteen years.

Wholeheartedly,

Angela

∾ ∾ ∾

November 23, 2009

I make the decision to invite my closest friends and colleagues at work to my classroom for a meeting this afternoon. In order to not clue them in to anything, I invite them through email first thing before school starts, explaining that the meeting will be at the end of the day. This way I can dodge a lot of the "What's going on, Angela?" questions for at least one full school day.

Our school is small enough that we are truly one big happy family, and like all families, we can be somewhat dysfunctional at times. Within five minutes of anything happening to anyone, the whole building knows, as if some silent alarm is set off in our hearts. Usually, every colleague knows when someone else goes home sick, is experiencing any type of crisis, or has had a bad bowel movement, for that matter. More importantly, I don't want to relive my same story fifteen or twenty times, retelling all of my coworkers in the hallways of our school and on the phone from home. I prefer to tell many friends and colleagues all at once, and to do it in the comfort of my classroom with Joe supporting me at my side.

So, the first thing I do when I enter my classroom in the morning is turn on my computer. My heart is pounding despite having done meditation earlier this morning, but I know this is a brave thing to do. It feels less important to be a private person right now and more important to be open. I type the email, take a deep breath, and hit "send."

Within minutes, the emails come pouring in and continue to do so all day. "Are you leaving us?" "Are you taking that sabbatical you wanted?" "Are you writing your third book?" "Are you going to work for your publisher?" Not one email reads, "Are you having a proactive mastectomy and hysterectomy to save your life?"

The buzz has started, but I quietly remain in my room. At lunchtime, I go for a walk to dodge any questions. Throughout the day I take deep breaths and focus on the children's lively energy and smiles. I feel scared the whole day, which is actually quite helpful because it continually keeps me in the moment.

After I line the children up to go home at dismissal time, I put them on their busses one by one, like picking the petals off a daisy, with "I love you, I love you too, I love you, I love you too . . ." I head back towards my classroom and use the bathroom before the meeting. My heart is pounding, just like earlier in the day, and I continue to use this as my metronome to life. It is my spirit pounding internally, cheering and shouting, "Way to go, Angela! You're making the best decision. I know it is hard to do but look at your growth!"

Everyone who enters my room is quiet. They each find a seat around my little pre-K tables. My friend Patty stands at the door, greeting everyone and keeping her eye on the hallway, waiting for Joe. Patty is one of my closest friends. She knows everything at this point. Patty is the school's physical education teacher and she gets along with everyone because everyone takes their students to the gym. She is upbeat and has become my dear confidant over the years. Ironically, I am the only teacher who doesn't take their students to the gym. But, somehow, we have connected on another level than merely as teachers; we've connected on a spiritual level.

My friends and colleagues continue to pile into the room and sit around the play kitchen furniture. Somehow, I know that a bit of information must have slipped out to them. I can feel their earnest solemnity. I don't feel upset that they know something already; I actually feel more relieved that Patty has probably warned them that there is something serious I need to discuss. Patty steps away from the doorway. "Here comes Joe," she announces.

I sit in the middle of the room looking at some notes I wrote down on an index card. I use the index cards because I know this is going to be emotional and I don't want to leave out anything that I feel needs to be shared. There is an empty chair next to me for Joe. As he enters the room, Joe apologizes for being late, which I think is very sweet since he is only late by three minutes. However, it does feel like twenty minutes due to the serious feeling in the room.

I begin by thanking everyone for coming and saying that what I want to share with them is difficult. I explain that it will be helpful if everyone can let me get through all the information from my index cards. I dance around the issue that I don't want people to interrupt and ask questions. Joe sits with his elbows on his knees, looking at his clasped hands, as if in prayer.

Just as I start to read from my index cards, I look over at one of my closest friends, Pam. We have been dear friends since the start of my career at CSCS. She has been another of my confidants through all of my decisions so far. I haven't even started to explain the nuts and bolts to the others and she is already crying. Pam has had more time to think about all my *BRCA1* information. Less than two weeks ago, we were eating wings at the Elbow Room bar after I had all my cancer tests at the Arnot Hospital. I am touched to see her get emotional.

I look back at my cards and start to discuss how it is very important for me to be genetically tested because my dad died of lung cancer at forty-two, his mom of breast cancer at forty-seven, my uncle of liver and colon cancer at fifty-eight, my mom of breast cancer at fifty-two, and her mom of uterine cancer at fifty-two. As I share this information from my index cards, I look up at everyone sitting around the tables and see my friend Nikki with tears in her eyes. I notice most people's jaws are slightly open, flabbergasted by my shocking familial history.

Next, I look carefully at my index card and notice that I have starred a reference point: Tell them about all the other cancer tests you've already had. I begin to cry, as if what I've been through is just now hitting me emotionally. It's because I have been so busy making appointments, going to appointments, researching, and making decisions that I haven't ever stopped to reflect on what I am going through.

I hold back my tears as I explain about *BRCA1* and that the doctors have had me go through some rigorous test these last two weeks.

I want everyone to know that, in this short time, I've had a mammogram, a CAT scan, a transvaginal ultrasound, X-rays, a CA125 blood test for ovarian cancer, and that I will have a colonoscopy next week. I want to inform them of all these tests because I need them to walk away from this meeting knowing one important fact: I do *not* have cancer.

I look up again at everyone and I am so pleased that no one has interrupted my train of thought; my friend Trecelle sits quietly, rocking herself back and forth. It was as if my friends and colleagues were in a *BRCA1* lesson for the day.

To wrap our meeting up I share the bigger news, as if everything I have just said isn't enough for everyone.

"With all this said, two weeks from now I will be having a preventative mastectomy, followed by a total hysterectomy in eight weeks. By doing these proactive surgeries, I reduce my chances of getting cancer by ninety percent."

Joe chimes in at this point. He looks up from his clasped hands and says, "You did good!" He smiles gravely at everyone. "We all need to support Angela and her decisions."

After Joe tells everyone that he appreciates their having come today, Patty makes a firm announcement. "So if anyone, teacher or community member, asks about Angela's health, you need to make sure you include that she DOES NOT have cancer."

Trecelle stops rocking and stands to hug me first. Joel stays sitting in disbelief. Heywood hugs me next and doesn't let go for some time. People are now lined up behind him for hugs as well. He whispers in my ear. "If you need anything at all, let me know. We can watch Adele."

I laugh and cry at the same time. "I'll be holding you to that promise." Then I punch his arm like a sister would do.

Heywood holds his arm like he's in pain and shouts. "Ouch!"

Some friends laugh at Heywood. There's no longer any tension in the air, only support and relief.

Everyone else hugs me before they leave as well. Joel doesn't move from his chair and waits there until only Patty, Pam, and Trecelle remain. Then he says, "I didn't like it that you said not to interrupt. I've wanted to hug you from the start of your story."

We hug, and Patty again makes sure that the last people at the meeting definitely know their facts. "If people ask, be sure to explain that Angela DOES NOT have cancer," she reminds them.

I love Patty. She makes sure that once any rumor starts flying around that no one gets that part wrong. I feel a sense of relief. Once everyone departs from my classroom, I gather my things and head for the parking lot. I get in my ol' gray Jeep Grand Cherokee and pat the steering wheel.

"Hang in there! I'm going to need you more than ever to cart my butt to all of these doctor's appointments."

I start my vehicle and the radio is playing Journey's "Anyway You Want It." I smile and think how appropriate it is.

When I pull in the driveway, Richard walks outside to help me carry things in.

"How did it go?" he immediately asks.

We kiss and I tell him how blessed I am by all the fine people in my life. Once inside, we immediately begin making dinner together. I uncork a bottle of Pinot Noir and start to tell him about my day.

Adele comes running through the kitchen. "What's for dinner, what's for dinner?"

I grab her to make her stop and hug me. She laughs and squirms to pull away from me. I give her a light spank.

"Spaghetti!" I say with a smile. "Please set the table."

I haven't told Adele any details yet, since she is only eight years old. However, when I do decide to tell her, I will focus mostly on that fact that she will be staying over at my friend Jennifer's house. I will make sure she knows that they get better cable channels than us and that Jennifer's daughters, Sabrina and Mayce, will be there with lots of fun and different toys. I will leave the adult issues of incisions, pain medications, and missing body parts to the adults.

After dinner, I take my dog Odie for a walk. I feel gratitude running through my blood that tomorrow is the last day of school before Thanksgiving vacation. I feel gratitude for not having cancer, for having great friends, colleagues to work with, a supportive husband, and two healthy children.

When I return from my walk, I get out my clothes for tomorrow's last workday. Fridays have traditionally been the time that we teachers all wear jeans. Even though tomorrow is Tuesday, it's virtually a Friday in the teaching world since it's the last day of the workweek before a vacation, making it a jeans day as well. I pull out my favorite jeans and a red T-shirt that simply reads INSPIRED! in large white letters.

As I set my clothes on my dresser, I do feel inspired. I feel like I am an inspiration. I have so many damn feelings running through every cell of my body right now that the words on my T-shirt feel like an understatement. I crawl into bed and lie on my clean, crisp sheets, shutting my eyes as gratitude smiles throughout my whole being.

∾ ∾ ∾

When I wake up at my usual 5:00 a.m. time, I sit with Richard in meditation. Somehow, being high on gratitude last night, followed by a run and a good night's sleep, has made me hungry for more goodness. Meditation seems like the perfect starting ingredient. When I sit, however, I observe uncomfortable feelings coming forth. I judge myself for choosing the INSPIRED! T-shirt. I ridicule myself and say the shirt should read, EXPOSED!

Throughout meditation, which is only twenty minutes long, I review the previous day's meeting and wonder if I gave too much information. I review, ruminate, review, ruminate. All of this is nothing new to me, however meditation usually brings me back to the present moment and helps me let go of all that nonsense. In today's meditation, I am aware of how long it is taking me to quiet my monkey mind.

In the middle of meditation, I focus more on something visual. I visualize a bright light swirling in my center and growing with each inhalation. As I exhale, I picture the light going to others in the world, especially those who have suffering in their lives. Inhaling, I see the light filling my whole body, and exhaling I send calming light to others. Inhaling, exhaling, and calming my mind are the antidotes for any ruminating thoughts. Richard gently taps me on my shoulder to let me know our twenty minutes are up. I decide to keep the red INSPIRED! T-shirt for today's work with a gentle, "You chose that for a reason, so go with it!" The T-shirt certainly goes with my life's current circumstances.

When I get to work, I walk to my mailbox, as I always do. However, this time the walk is different. As I look at everyone else, I can see sympathy in their eyes. I can tell the news has spread already and I am back to my EXPOSED! feeling.

The first friendly face that I see is Joe. I greet him the way I always do.

"Hey, boss!"

He looks down with a smile, as if it is hard for him to take me calling him "boss."

"How you doing?" he asks.

"I'm okay, just feeling more 'exposed' than 'inspired.'"

"You can be everything!" he offers.

His simple words are enough to transform me again. I smile and continue onward. I love it that one person's words can mean so much. I feel better, and this sets the tone for my day.

I have a week and a half until my mastectomy. First things first, however. Wednesday is my colonoscopy, and Thursday is Thanksgiving. When people stop me in the hallway to ask how I am doing, I tell them I am feeling great but the doctor wants me to get this one last cancer screening out of the way before my mastectomy. I jokingly mention that I have to fast two days before Thanksgiving and I will have my colonoscopy the day before the holiday. I laugh harder that I will be able to stuff myself even more with turkey and pie because I will have flushed out everything beforehand. Older teachers who have had colonoscopies are able to connect with me and talk about the chalky drink, which, according to them, is the worst thing about the whole process. Because I have never actually had a colonoscopy, I'm not sure if I should agree with this. In my mind, I am certain that a chalky drink is better than a camera hose up my butt. Nonetheless, I am soon to find out.

～ ～ ～

School is now on vacation for the Thanksgiving holiday. The night before my colonoscopy, I prepare myself by fasting, which I find is not such a big deal. The only problem I have with the fasting is that I am asked to not drink red wine. And I love my red wine! So, I suffer through a white wine evening instead. The nurse has told me that red wine, or any purple juices for that matter, can cause coloring in the colon that can be misinterpreted during the procedure, so white wine is the only option. Then, the chalky drink comes into play. I hadn't realized it was more than one chalky drink. My night becomes one chalky drink after another, and another, and another. There's an ungodly amount of water to drink and it keeps me running to the bathroom all night.

It's so bad that I actually have to remove myself from our bedroom. I go to sleep on the downstairs couch because I get up so frequently that I am keeping my husband awake. I try to rest on the couch, but continue to run to the downstairs bathroom, then back to the couch, then back to the bathroom, then back to the couch. This happens so much that I don't even make it back to the couch. I now rest at the kitchen counter in between my bodily explosions. Sitting on the kitchen stool, I lay my sweaty head on my clammy arms and drape my upper body over the whole kitchen countertop. Much of my long curly hair is over my sweaty face, and I feel my mom's spunk in me as I blurt out, "There has got to be a better frickin' way to prep for a colonoscopy. It's frickin' 2009, for God's sake! Isn't there a pill or something you can take?"

I run to the bathroom again. When Richard comes down stairs to make coffee at 5 a.m., I am still up and in the "prep process." We have to leave by 7 a.m. for the hospital and I keep my spirits up by joking with him.

"I hope I don't poop my pants in the car before I get there."

"I'm sure the nurses have seen it all," Richard assures me, "so don't worry."

I make it to the hospital with clean underwear and all. I am starving and assure the nurse at check-in that I am all scoured out. She laughs even though she has probably heard that joke a hundred times this month. She tells Richard that she will come and get him when I am finished, at which point we can talk with the doctor. Richard and I give each other a peck.

I feel good with this nurse. She smiles when I tell her I like her glasses.

She points to mine. "I was thinking that about yours."

She is a woman in her later fifties, looking well put together in her nurse scrubs and perfect makeup. If I were flipping through a nurse catalog and had to pick scrubs to wear to work, I think I'd choose exactly what she has on today. She looks very yoga-like in her uniform. Her top is a traditional nurse top but it ties in the back and is a pretty lavender India print. Her shoes look extremely comfortable, expensive, and classy, the kind that you could wear all day. I hope I look as good as she does when I get to be in my fifties. Her nametag reads NELL.

She gives me a gown and tells me everything should come off, with the gown opening in the back. I bravely try not to think about why the opening has to be in the back. While I lie down on the gurney, Nell looks over my paperwork. "Are you having medical problems, is that why you are here today? Why are you having a colonoscopy at your young age?"

I tell Nell everything I know about BRCA and her jaw opens in disbelief after I explain my genetic test results.

"They actually know those numbers?" she asks in amazement.

In my mind, I can't believe that I, a teacher, know more about *BRCA1* than the nurse in front of me. I begin to tell her all the statistics.

Nell sets her clipboard down and walks over as if she wants to hug me but instead pulls the sheet up to my shoulders. "I'm so sorry you have to go through all of this. I'm going to take good care of you today. Can I give you some relaxant medication?"

"Do you think I'll need it?" I ask her.

"Oh, this will only mellow you out before you get the real medication."

It's as if Nell has asked to buy me a drink at the bar, and I take her up on it. "Sure," I shrug. I think, *What the heck, a little buzz before a hose goes up my butt would probably be good for me.*

Nell comes back and shoots something into my IV, and I instantly feel high. But it makes me teary-eyed. I feel so naked and vulnerable on the gurney, high and listless. Nell hugs me and I whisper, "I miss my mom!"

She then gives me Versed, a sedative. Once injected, I feel an instantaneous rush of reassurance and comfort, and for a nanosecond I understand why people become addicted.

The next thing I know, Nell is wiping my hair away from my eyes. "We're taking you to the operating room now." Once I'm wheeled into the cold room, Dr. Miller says he needs me to roll on my side. All I feel is the scope being injected and I cry out. "Oh!"

The last thing I remember is Dr. Miller saying, "Give her more medicine."

When I come to, Nell is standing by my bedside with a little pint of OJ and a piece of wheat toast. She tells me I did good and that she is proud of me. She is going to get my husband and he can help me get dressed. I wish she could come home with me and be my mom.

When Richard comes into the room he gives me a "Hellooooo!" I am behind the curtain and I'm already getting ready to leave. As I balance on one leg, trying to put my foot in the other pant leg, he rushes over. "Whoa, easy, let me help you."

I am still higher than a kite and probably higher than usual because of the extra dosage. It feels good letting Richard help me. He even ties my shoes. Nell comes in soon after and says that Dr. Miller is ready to talk with us.

Richard and I walk arm in arm into a very busy area. I am immediately aware of the awkwardness of the area as it doesn't seem like a place you would talk to a doctor. Dr. Miller is in front of a computer on one side of a hallway area and we are sitting on the other side of the hallway. Nurses and other hospital staff walk between us as we discuss the results from my colonoscopy.

I already know the results have to be okay, even in the state of euphoria that I am coming down from, because no doctor in their right mind would deliver bad news in such a public setting. Or, at least I hope they wouldn't.

The exit door is less than four feet away from my right and I see it swing open and shut with each hospital staff member who passes through it. I think to myself that it should have a sign on it that reads, QUICK! GET YOUR BUTT OUT OF HERE SO WE CAN GET TO OUR NEXT COLONOSCOPY. The workers are casually walking between our conversation, never saying excuse me, just carrying on like we are invisible. Had I received a hospital survey about my hospital experience, I would have shared that normal people like to talk about their colonoscopies in a private office. But I am never asked to fill one out.

～ ～ ～

The next day is Thanksgiving and it is the first one in years that I don't cook and entertain a houseful of people. Instead, we go to my brother- and sister-in-law's home for a quiet dinner. After we eat, Adele scurries off to go play on the computer, while Matthew goes to the basement to fiddle with the guitars in my brother-in-law's recording area. Richard and Gary clean up and talk in the kitchen while my sister-in-law, Melissa, and I drink wine in the living room.

We sit on the couch facing each other, each with one bare foot tucked under ourselves. Melissa has kidney dialysis four times a week and has been mostly concerned with her diabetic condition and the aches and pains that she deals with daily.

"Angela, I'm in awe of you.," Melissa says as she sips her wine. "I just can't believe how brave you are."

"Brave? Look at you and what you have to cope with on a daily basis! You're the brave one!" I counter, and then sip some red wine.

Melissa shakes her head. "No, you're the brave one. My condition is chronic, yours is acute." She sips more wine. "I don't know if I could do what you're doing!"

"Oh God, yes you could!" I retort.

"Gary, bring us more wine!" Melissa suddenly yells out.

"You've already finished the bottle!" Gary shouts back.

"Well then, open another one," Melissa demands.

Soon after, Gary comes into the living room and fills up our glasses. We clink them together and I say, "Nostrovia."

Melissa slurs out "Nostrovia" in her best drunk Polish accent. "I'm so glad you're my sister-in-law. I love you, sister!"

8

Surgery and Pain (Meds)

December 2, 2009

Today is my last day of school before my first operation. At the beginning of the day I find two presents on my desk. The first is a pair of ivory slippers from Gwen. The other is from my assistant and is a green robe with ivory stars on it. Later, Sherry delivers a third present to my room: green and ivory pajamas. I love it that the three of them created the coziest gift for my recovery. I tell them that I am going to be the coziest, most stylish recovery woman for the next six weeks.

At the end of the day, many of my best friends wander into my room, not saying much of anything. Just their presence touches my heart, though. Heywood walks in with his hands in his pocket and Patty tells him to quit playing with himself. He pulls out one hand from his pocket and flips her off. Joel and Pam laugh. I laugh and become teary-eyed at the same time. "I love you guys!"

Heywood gives me a hug. "If you need anything, anything at all, just give me a call. We'd love to have Adele over for a night or two."

I hug Heywood back. "I was going to take you up on your offer."

"You better," he says.

Joel hugs me too. "I love you Fish!"

I smile at Joel. "Richard will be calling Patty to let everyone know how I am doing."

"He better call me!" Joel says with a smile.

After the guys leave, I walk over to my desk and pull out my gift bag. I tell Pam, Patty, Sherry, and Doris, "I got presents for you too—Christmas presents!"

"Gee, you're having surgery tomorrow and thinking about Christmas presents for us? You should be thinking about you!" Sherry says.

Patty backs me up. "Let her do this! It makes her feel good."

It does make me feel good. I hand everyone the same-sized jewelry box and tell them to open them at once because they're all the same. As they do, I am still teary-eyed. I got them all the circular, pink rhinestone necklaces back in mid-November when I went for my marathon of cancer tests. Each one has a breast cancer emblem and a poem about hope.

"Oh, I love it," Pam says first.

"Oh yes, it's beautiful," Doris chimes in, while Patty says they will all wear them tomorrow for my surgery day. Before they leave I hug the four of them, explaining that I have to get home because I haven't done anything to get ready for tomorrow.

Just before I lock my door to leave, the classroom phone rings. I think this is odd because I've already spoken with all my friends. I notice that the caller ID says its the principal from the high school. She is not only the principal, but I have her daughter as a student in my pre-K classroom. I like her because she truly appreciates my work with little ones. I answer the phone with my upbeat spirit.

"Hey you!" Lisa says, relieved. "I'm so glad I caught you before you left. I just want you to know that I'm sending you an angel tomorrow."

"What?" I say, unsure of what she means.

"My mom is a nurse at Robert Packer Hospital, and she'll be working there when you get there. I told her you were coming and to take good care of you."

I smile and feel the warmth from all the love in my life. "Thanks Lisa! *You're* an angel!"

Before I walk out the door for my six week departure, I glance over at my plans for the substitute teacher. "Good luck!" I murmur.

~ ~ ~

December 3, 2009

The drive to Robert Packer Hospital takes nearly an hour and a half. When Richard and I finally arrive, we offhandedly joke about our extreme promptness and how we are so happy to be on time to now sit and wait. Once we are in the waiting area, I check in with the receptionist.

She takes my name and date of birth, points out where the bathrooms are, and tells me that someone will be with me shortly. I have worn my comfortable yoga clothes, and Richard is wearing his soft flannel shirt and black fleece vest that he wears most of the week at home. I rest my head on his velvety shoulder and smell the familiar fabric softener I use in our wash. I even smell a hint of his shaving lotion that he used the night before. Richard represents the solid strength of home and hearth and comfort to me, all of which are needed at this very moment.

A man walks by with a coffee and Danish. Richard twists his head to see where he is coming from and then notices a small back table in the waiting area with free coffee and Danishes. He kisses my forehead and tells me he will wait until they take me in before he has any. He knows I have been fasting since midnight.

At that moment, and to my surprise right on schedule, a nurse walks out through the double doors with a clipboard and looks around the waiting area.

"Angela?" she calls out.

I raise my hand quietly so she notices me, handing my purse, phone, and all of my belongings to my husband.

"Keep track of all of this," I tell him.

Richard takes his focus off the coffee and sweets and kisses me. "I'm keeping track of you!"

We kiss again, then again, and say "I love you" more than once.

I take only my anxiety with me as I walk with the nurse down a long hallway, and we make small talk to keep my angst smaller than my bravery. "So, how long have you worked here?" I ask.

As she shares about herself, I hear nothing. My focus is on the floors, the germ-free, sterile hallway which holds nothing; no table with magazines, no lamp, no pictures, nothing. It is just a long sanitized walkway painted a clean pale yellow. The only comfort I feel is from the fact that it's disinfected.

As we near the end of the foyer, I feel the coldness of the operating room in the air. It probably feels cooler to me since I haven't had any food or drink since midnight. The nurse presses a button and the double door opens up with a gust of chilliness. It is as if she opened the doors to Oz and the workers are seen rushing and dancing around as they work.

This is the cold and busy holding and preparation space for everyone having surgery this morning. There are fifteen to twenty prep stations partitioned with curtains and people in scrubs are busily running from one station to the next. I get the feeling of being at a horse race: "And they're off! Angela Schmidt Fishbaugh is in the lead with a full mastectomy followed by Jane Doe who will be having hernia surgery."

The nurse points to a partition. "We're going to curtain number five." She pulls it open to show me my area where a folded gown and white sheet are on the gurney. She hands me a flimsy blue zipper bag, telling me that all my personal belongings and clothes will go in there and that the bag will be returned to me after surgery.

Everything is said in a very matter-of-fact fashion, as if this is the hundredth time she has repeated these words this week. She points to the gown on the gurney and, without looking at me, asks me to get undressed and put on the gown, opening to the front.

Her telling me to get undressed reminds me of my purple-marked breasts and I'm suddenly acutely aware of the actual operation that is going to take place within the hour. As I begin to take off my clothes I remember my pockets are empty. *Oh no*, I think anxiously. My chapstick is in my purse and my mind is now racing about how to get it back.

I put all my belongings in the blue bag and lie down on the narrow wheeled bed. My lips feel dry, and all I can think about is how I can score some chapstick. This has been an issue for me for years. Ever since I stopped smoking in 1996 I have had tubes stashed here and there like a typical addict. They are in my purse, by my night stand, and in my car. I also have a stash in my desk at work. Even when I was delivering my daughter, dilated 10 cm and in excruciating pain, I was *still* slathering my lips with it. I wonder how I am going to make it from surgery to post surgery and then to recovery without my chapstick.

"Hello!" I hear from behind my curtain. When it opens I notice it is Lisa's mother. I remember her right away from when she came to a special pre-K event for her granddaughter.

"How are you doing?" she asks sweetly.

I immediately start to cry. "I left my chapstick with Richard in the waiting room."

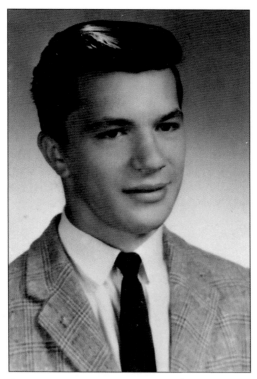

Dad's graduation picture – 1965

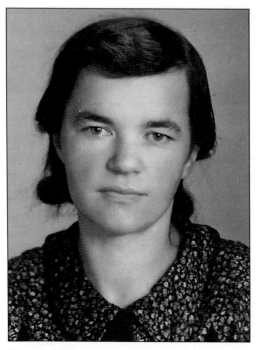

Grandma Schmidt – 1949

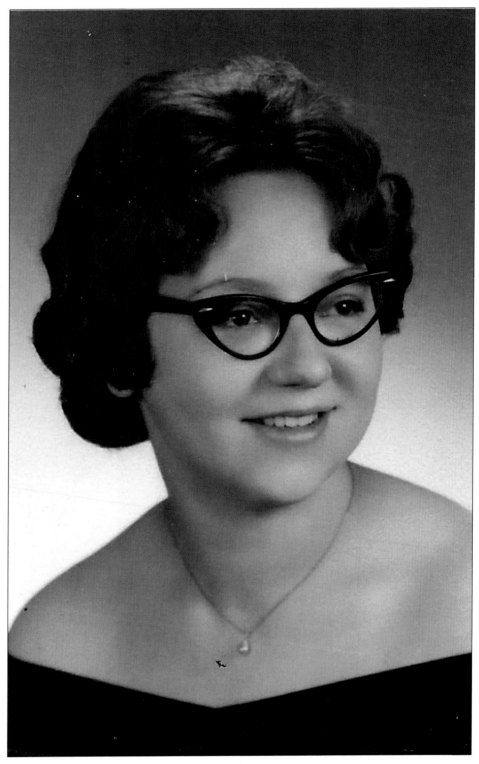

Godmother's graduation picture – 1965

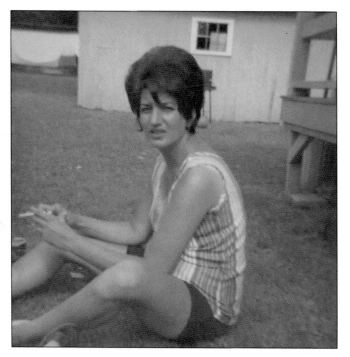

Mom in the backyard – 1973

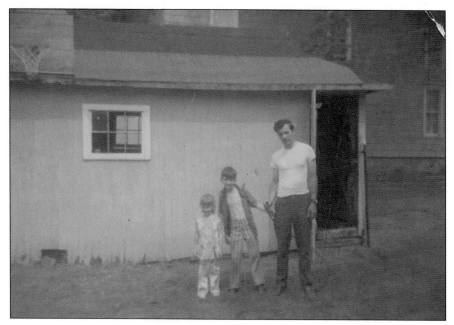

Angela, brother Ben, and Dad – June 1973

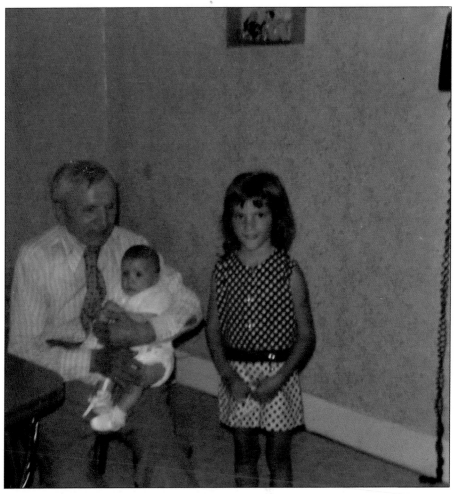

Angela at home with Grandpa and sibling – 1973

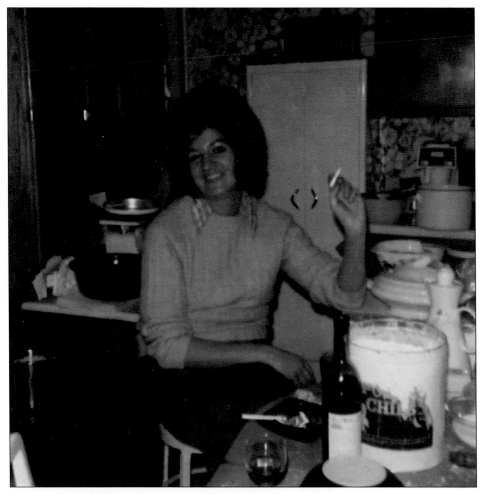

Mom cooking at the home of Angela's godmother

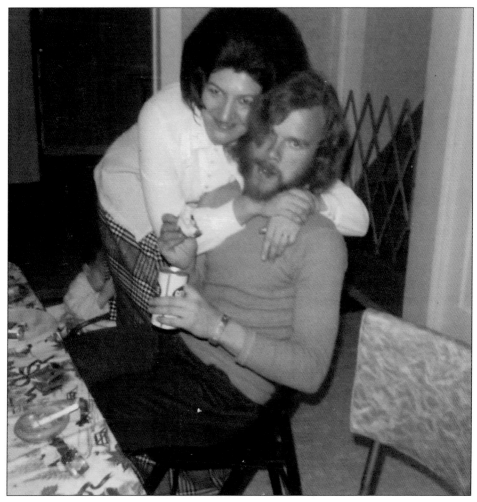

Mom and Uncle John after his return from Vietnam – 1974

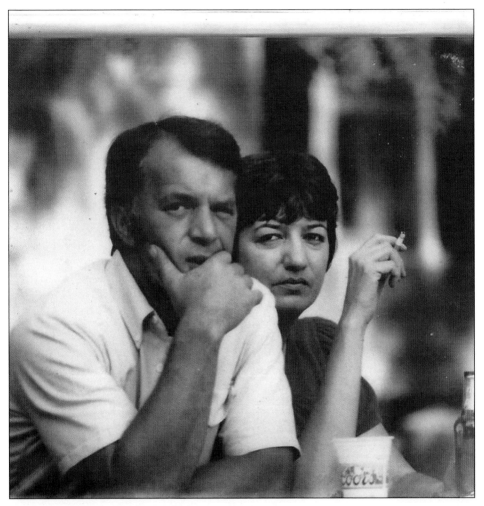

Stanley and Marlene – June 1986

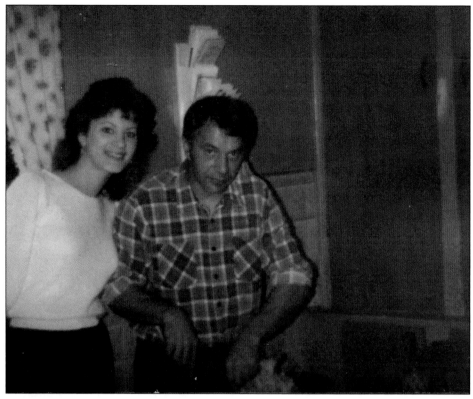

Angela and her dad – Thanksgiving Day, 1986

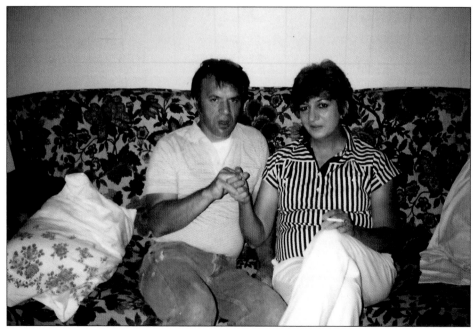

Dad home for a weekend visit from the psychiatric ward – late summer, 1987

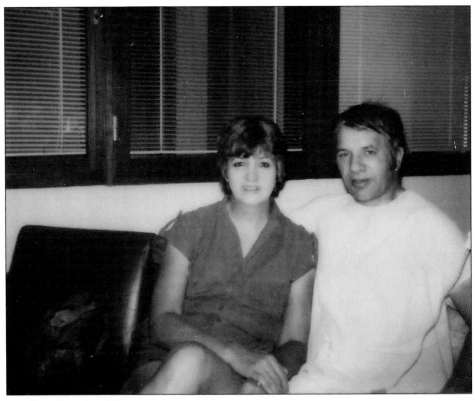

Dad's first month of chemotherapy treatment – October 1987

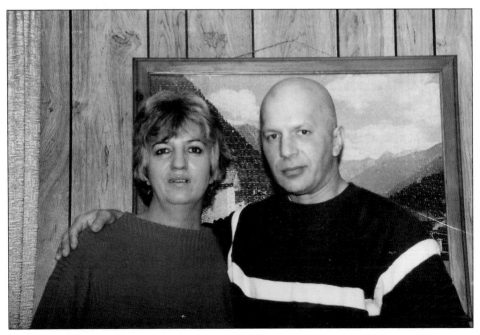

Dad and Mom – December 1987

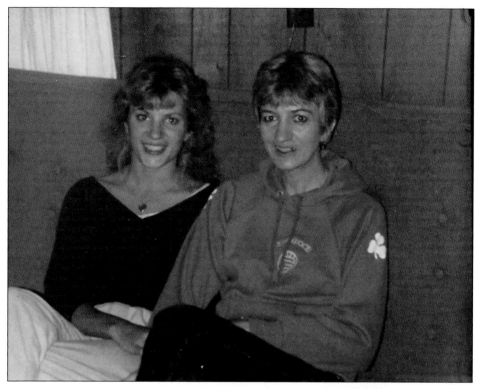

Angela and her mom, two months after Dad's death – October 1988

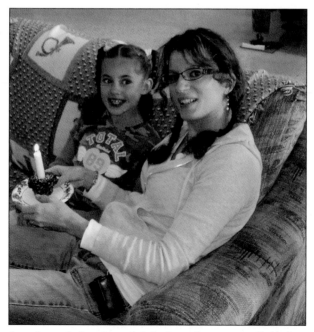

Angela and daughter Adele less than a month before Angela's first surgery

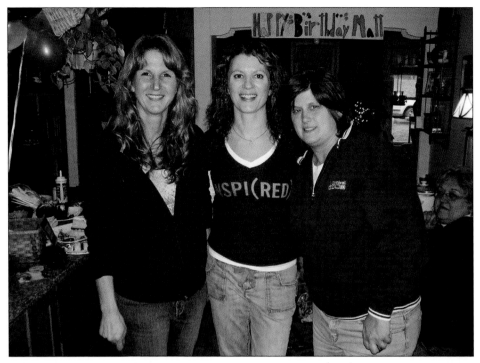

Angela with her two oldest friends (Maureen at left, Cheryl at right), just five days before Angela's first surgery

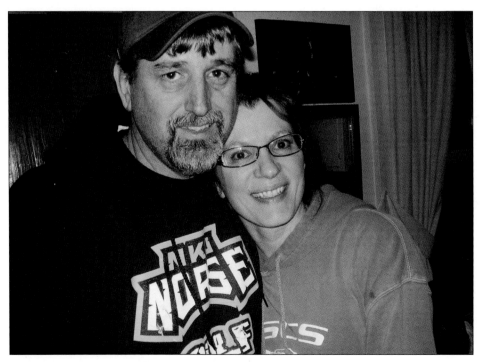

Angela with her brother Ben after her hysterectomy

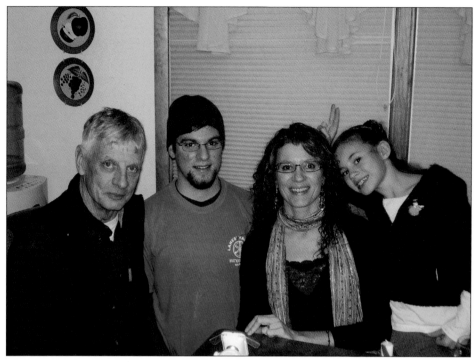

The family at Angela's godmother's for Christmas, just two weeks after mastectomy –
December 2009

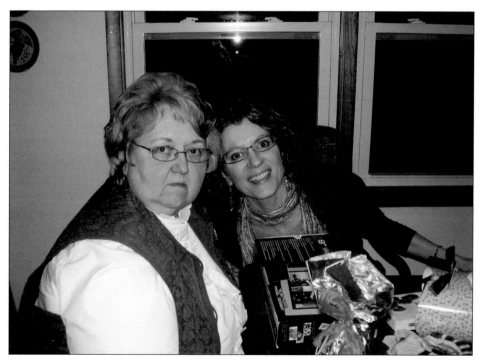

Angela and Godmother after the mastectomy – Christmas 2009

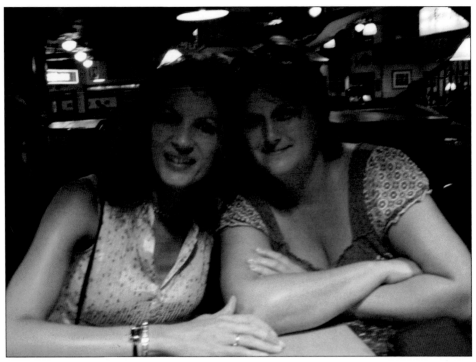

Angela and oldest friend Cheryl after Angela's reconstructive surgery – Summer 2010

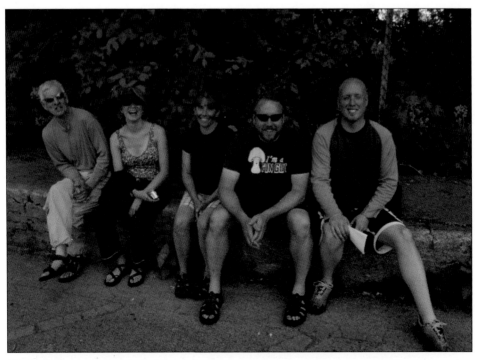

Richard, Angela, and their friends before whitewater rafting down the Black River in Upstate New York

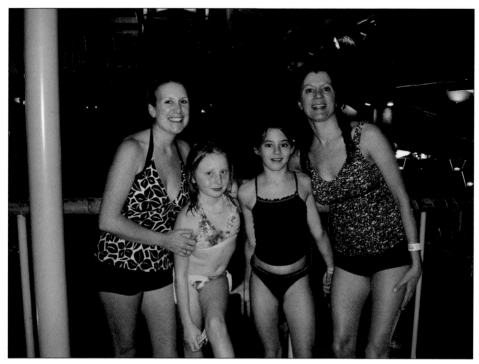

At Splash Lagoon after going down Hurricane Hole

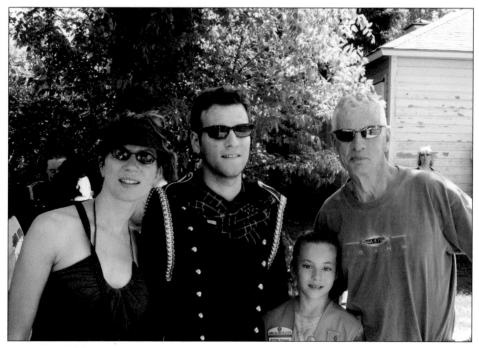

One month after last surgery – Memorial Day, 2010

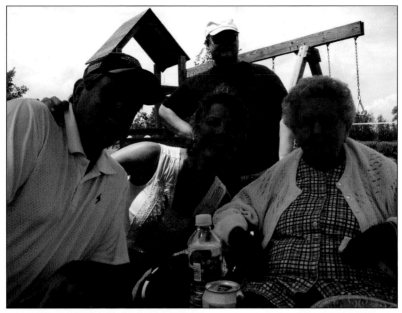

After all the surgeries: Brother Ben, Angela, Godmother's mom Genny, and Godmother's husband Bob (in back) – June 2010

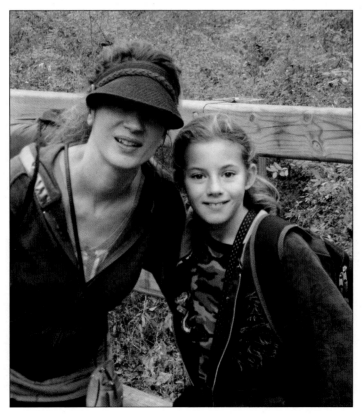

After all the surgeries: Angela hiking with her daughter Adele

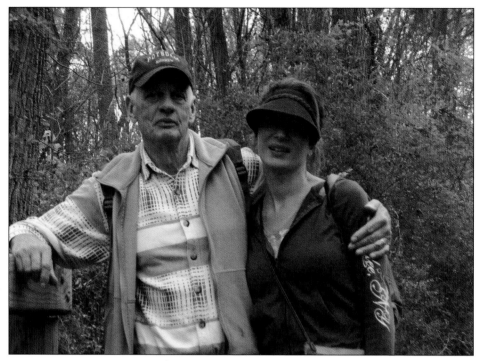

After all the surgeries: Angela hiking with her husband Richard

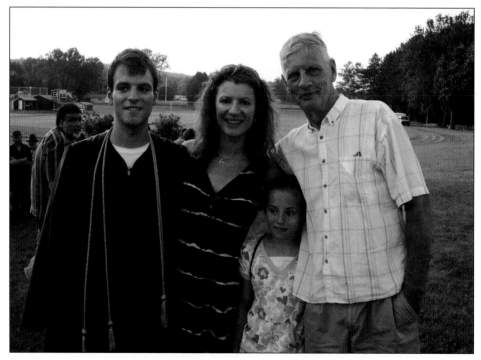

The family

"Don't cry," she says. "I'll take care of this." She swipes my hair from my forehead and gently tucks it behind my ear. "I'll be right back," she says as she leaves, closing the curtain behind her.

When she returns, she says hello again and then opens the curtain. "I have something better than chapstick."

Standing with her is Richard. I start to cry and smile. "You *are* an angel! I didn't know Richard could come back here!"

"We don't advertise it, I'm not sure why. I think immediate family should be able to come back here. Sometimes there are too many members though. You two take some time together." Then she shuts the curtain behind her to give us some privacy.

Richard kisses me and I see he's teary-eyed too. He takes my chapstick out of his pocket, swirls it around my lips, and then kisses me again.

"I'm sorry," I say, mostly apologizing for not keeping my emotions perfectly in check.

"Shhh," Richard consoles, kissing me again and then placing his body so he's half sitting and half lying on the waiting table with me. His head rests on my shoulder and I stroke his hair.

Dr. Panilio now enters through the curtain without as much as a hello. He asks, in his Filipino accent, "How are you today?" However, once he actually sees my tears, he can tell that I am an emotional piece of baggage, ready to be lugged to the operating room.

"I'm okay," I say, starting to get teary-eyed and apologetic again. My apologies are for, well, for having emotions in the first place.

He nods and opens my gown to look at his purple markings on my small breasts.

"I did a good job of not getting the skin tape wet in my bath this morning, didn't I?" I say to him.

He smiles. "Very good!"

When the nurse comes in to check my IV, he instructs her to give me something for "this," pointing to my tears. She asks how much and he orders the maximum dosage. Dr. Panilio's take-charge demeanor helps stabilize my emotions.

"Don't worry. I make you look good in bathing suit," he says to me as he closes my gown.

I nod, taken aback by this comment about a bathing suit. My body is being cut up this morning. I'm not at all concerned about a bathing suit!

After Dr. Panilio leaves, I look up at Richard. He reads my mind about the bathing suit comment and rolls his eyes.

"Let it go," he says. "Dr. Panilio must think that every American woman's only concern is to look good in a bathing suit."

The nurse comes in with the medication and inserts it into my IV. And oh my! Within seconds every cell of my body is high. All my bad feelings disappear. It feels like each blood cell is floating, with no cares in the world, and I let go and am no longer in control of anything. I reach my hand up towards Richard and slur, "Baby, can I have my chapstick?"

"They're ready for you, Angela," the nurse interrupts. "Richard, we'll call you immediately when she is out of the operating room. It should be before lunchtime."

Richard kisses my woozy smile and then my head rocks back and forth. I feel like singing Stevie Wonder's "You Are the Sunshine of My Life."

The journey to the operating room feels long and dreamy. When the medical gang pushes me through into the operating room, I find that there are numerous surgeons, five of which are Dr. Gioe's top residents, all ready to learn from Robert Packer Hospital's king of surgery. It's like a party, with classic rock music playing in the background, but instead of a disco ball, there are beautiful, state of the art operating room lights.

The anesthesiologist gets down in my face. "Are you doing okay, Angela?"

My drunken "uh-huh" is good enough for her. "Okay Angela, we're going to give you anesthesia and when you wake up you'll be in recovery." The oxygen mask then goes over my face.

If my family had had more money, my mom would have ended up looking like Joan Rivers or Dolly Parton or Michael Jackson. She was that type of surgery addict. Mom had gall bladder surgery, a hysterectomy, an ulcer surgery, and a partial mastectomy. I'm certain she would have had plastic surgery had my dad not gambled all his money away.

Before coming home from the hospitals, she always managed to shake down the doctors for every prescription she could get. Oh, and also before every surgery too. Before each visit, the nurses and doctors would tell her to wash all her makeup off, to shampoo her hair, and not use any hairspray. But my mom always showed up to her surgeries with the same makeup and teased hair. She said that if those top paid nurses and doctors didn't want her to have makeup and hairspray on, then they could take it off themselves. That's what she was paying them for.

In preparing, Mom would lick her Maybelline black eyeliner pencil—saying that it went on smoother when she did that—then outline her eyebrows. She'd also cover her eyelids with the same eyeliner. Not just a line though. Rather, completely cover the entire lid of her eye. She wore black mascara too, everyday. Underneath it all was a thick layer of cream foundation, one shade darker than her tanning bed skin, and she always had a makeup line underneath her jaw bone.

She smoked a cigarette while she styled her hair, even when she sprayed a quarter of an Aqua Net aerosol can. Everyone in our family joked that Mom was going to die in one of two ways. The first way of death was by blowing herself up in the bathroom while doing her hair and makeup. The second way was by burning up in the recliner, because she passed out each evening with a lit cigarette in her hand. Sometimes the long ash would drop and leave burn marks on her housecoat.

Unsurprisingly, my mom's hair never moved, even in her red convertible car or fishing boat. When the nurses would try to wash her makeup off, the eye-lined brows still remained, as if she had permanently dyed that area of her skin from years of using a Maybelline pencil. My mom also had false teeth. She demanded that she be able to keep them in her mouth until the last second, just before taking her to surgery. And when they did remove her teeth, she'd say the same thing to me, right before they whisked her away: "If anything happens to me, the tin box is in my closet at home."

I had been hearing about the tin box since I was a little girl. I never actually saw what was in it, but I knew that whatever was in there had to be very important. As I got older, I'd finish her sentence for her before they wheeled her to the operating room.

"If anything happens to me—"

I'd finish it with a kiss to her forehead. "Yeah, yeah, the tin box is in your closet. Nothing is going to happen to you." Sometimes I joked and told her she didn't put enough Aqua Net hairspray on for the day's surgery.

When I come to from my mastectomy, I am in another waiting area with lots of curtains and stalls. While it's warmer than the original prep area, I'm still cold.

"How are you doing, Angela?" a nurse suddenly asks me.

"I'm thirsty," I say, clicking my tongue several times to the roof of my mouth to prove it.

"I can only get you some ice chips," the nurse responds in a bubbly tone.

Irritated by her response, I murmur, "Whatever you can do, please."

She leaves my area, and when she comes back she hands me a Styrofoam cup with ice chips and a plastic spoon.

"Can I have my blue bag with my personal stuff in it?" I ask the nurse.

"It's waiting for you in your room," she says sweetly. "We'll move you there soon. Your husband can meet you there too."

The wait seems long and I can see other people who have just had surgery on the other side of the room. There is a woman in front of me who appears to have gauze and bandages around her knee. There is a man to the right of her whose leg is in a cast and is raised up in a sling. Our eyes all meet, but we're all coming down from our medication high, so we don't say anything. There is no greeting, no waving; just our cold brave eyes as we come back to reality. I feel hazy, mystified, and powerless. It is heartbreaking to look at their weary bodies and know that I probably look worse.

Never having had a major surgery before, this is all a strange and unusual experience for me. I lift my sore left hand, the hand with the IV poking in it, and peek under the sheet to see if I can glimpse any sign of the surgery. I am scared that the IV might pull out, so I only use my left hand to slightly hold the blanket and sheet up. I carefully use my right hand to open my hospital gown, only to find—and now feel— that my chest area is firmly wrapped in white gauze, pins and tubes protruding from either side. My body is exhausted and I can't hold the blanket up any longer, so I allow my arms to collapse and close my eyes.

I remembered my mom coming home from her mastectomy. She came to stay at my home when she was released from the hospital. I took the day off from work and cared for her. I think it was actually the longest time she went without smoking since she was sixteen years old. She stopped for two whole days: the day she recovered in the hospital and the day she stayed in my home. I made pancakes for her and sat on the edge of the bed to feed her.

"Here, Mom!" I held up a syrupy bite to her drowsy face. "You should eat something."

"Thank you!" She took a bite then added, "You're my angel from heaven!"

I gave her another bite. "Mom, you really should stop smoking and start taking care of yourself better."

She smiled and winked at me. "I did stop smoking. I haven't smoked for two days."

"Yeah, I know. That's good!" I took a bite of her pancakes, then paused and said to her sadly, "You have cancer, so when you go home to your own place, you should quit smoking for good. And quit drinking that vodka crap too. Maybe try having just a glass or two of red wine."

Mom tapped my knee and looked despondently back in my eyes, "I miss our daddy!" She pointed to her purse and looked in pain as she held her chest. "Grab some pain medicine from my purse."

"I miss Dad too!" I wiped a tear away. "We all want you around for a long time, Mom. Okay?" I grabbed her purse but before handing it to her I wanted to make sure she heard me. "Okay?"

"Okay!" She half smiled, then shuffled through her large purse and pulled out her newest prescription bottle.

I felt extreme gratitude in my heart for having had that precious time to feed my mom pancakes, express our sadness together about missing Dad, and voice my opinion about her unhealthy lifestyle.

When I wake up, my mouth is still so dry that I can't even call out to the nurse to ask for a drink. When she does catch my eye, she comes over to pull the sheet up.

"Are you still doing okay, Angela?"

"I'm cold and I need more to drink," I say to her again.

"Honey, I still can't get you water. I'll bring you some more ice chips and another blanket," she responds.

When the nurse returns, she has a pillow under her arm, another flimsy white mesh blanket, and the small plastic cup filled with ice chips. She props me up with the pillow and feeds me an ice chip. I devour it and say "more," then devour another, and another.

"Can I have some medicine?" I ask her, when I finally feel hydrated.

"Are you in pain?" she asks me.

I fume a bit and spout off "I just had a mastectomy."

"On a scale of one to ten, ten being the highest, what is your pain?"

Truthfully, I have no idea. I roll my eyes upward as if I am looking into my mind to gauge the pain. I'm thinking, *I just had a mastectomy. I'm aching, I'm cold, thirsty, hungry, and I don't have warm bedding. I'm not allowed to drink or eat. So, tell the nurse something above a five.* I tell her my pain is a six.

The nurse brings a syringe after I tell her this and inserts it into my IV.

"What are you giving me?" I ask her.

"It's Norco."

I now feel the Norco running through my veins. My body feels heavy, lifeless, and carefree. I smile across the recovery room at my fellow recovery-room mates and close my eyes. The gal gives me a listless wave and I smile back a bigger smile but I'm too high to wave back.

My mom always had medication on her. It was in her purse, on the nightstand, in the medicine cabinet, in the top kitchen cupboard, and by the coffee maker. Whenever we went out anywhere, if she had to set her purse down or look for keys or anything of that nature, I could hear the pills shaking in their bottles.

"What the hell you got in there, Mom?" I'd ask her, jokingly.

Her response was usually a smoker's laugh and "Whatever you want." She would then begin to rant about her medications.

"For God's sake, it is 1986," she would say, the year changing to 1994, 1998, 1999, and 2000 as time went on. "There is no reason why anyone should have pain." Oftentimes the rant ended with, "My nerves are shot. I need a Valium." She'd then reach in her purse and pull out one of her many bottles and pop a few pills. Her persistent ranting would then mellow into slurry phrases like "bring me ashtray" or "light my cigarette sweetie, use the stove, I can't find my lighter." Or, if I tried to talk seriously about her health she'd say, "I'm not bothering anybody, just leave me alone."

I was thoroughly embarrassed by her use of drugs but I somehow came to accept it. Well, not entirely. My mom was not shy about discussing her love of drugs; how can anyone ever accept that? Mostly, I liked to offhandedly joke about it with my family, laugh about it with my friends, and basically hide it from the remainder of the world.

I'm woken by the familiar nurse standing by my bed, who now has a young man with her.

"Angela, we're going to take you up to your room now," she says. "Your husband will be there waiting for you."

"Can I eat?"

The young man, who is part of the evening shift, jumps in and offers to help. "Do you want me to get you a menu from the cafeteria? We can order it ahead of time."

"Uh-huh!" I nod.

"What would you like me to order?" he asks.

"Just food!" I slur, trying not to fade out as they begin to wheel my gurney down a long hallway.

Lying in the gurney and being carried away in snuggly wrapped blankets reminds me of how I would pretend to be sleeping on the couch and not wake up when my dad tried to say it was time for bed. He would then carry me upstairs while I'd keep my eyes closed. I felt safe knowing my dad was carrying me, even on our steep staircase. He would tuck me in and then head back downstairs to carry up my younger brother and sister. Sometimes he would even have to carry my mom to bed.

I keep my eyes shut and can now feel the Norco in full effect. It's at this very moment of complete release that the one small part of my brain that originally had anxiety, whispers, "Wow! I was really worried, and now I'm dreamy and relaxed. Relaxing feels so good, something I rarely get to do. Thanks, Norco!"

My husband is out in the hallway and follows them in with my bag of belongings. He waits outside the room until they are finished moving me to the hospital bed, where I discover that I have a catheter inserted into me along with all the other tubes. I begin pulling on it and ask, in my Norco way, "Hey, what's this?"

The nurse quickly taps my hand, just like you would instinctively slap a toddler's hand who is reaching for a light socket.

"No, no, no! Don't touch. That's your catheter."

"How long does that have to stay in there?"

"Until you can get up and go to the bathroom by yourself," she responds.

I assure her I can, but she states that she has to ask the doctor first. Once she is convinced I won't pull out any tubes or touch any more of the equipment, she tells my husband that he can come in to see me. She then leaves him in charge, explaining how the catheter and all the other tubes need to remain in place until she returns.

Although I'm famished, my attention is still focused on the uncomfortable feeling of the catheter in my private area and the IV in my hand, which feels like it is shooting into my bone rather than any vein. I am also focused on the tornado tubes that are holding the drainage liquid from my chest region. These tubes are literally safety pinned to white gauze underneath my hospital gown.

When the nurse's assistant appears, she is carrying a little mini golf pencil and a menu. I notice all of her tattoos and I can smell that she has recently smoked a cigarette. Her hospital scrubs have Betty Boop all over them. She hands me a small paper menu. "Here you go, Angela. Just check the boxes of what you would like to eat for your next three meals."

I realize again that my entire stay at the hospital is only one measly day, which includes three measly meals. As I check the boxes, I complain.

"Way back when I made my decision to have this operation, I was told I would only stay one night." I begin checking what sounds good: for breakfast, cranberry juice, coffee, toast, eggs; for lunch, roast pork, mashed potatoes, and carrots. I check everything there is for dinner and then tell the assistant what the doctor had said to me way back then. "Yeah, the doctor shared that they had an eighty-nine-year-old woman who had a mastectomy here last week, and she only stayed one night."

The nursing assistant shakes her head judgmentally, knowing exactly why I am irritable. "I know it. Isn't that awful?" she agrees.

I hand her back the paper and preach to the choir some more. "Yeah, I even said to him, 'Just because an eighty-nine-year-old goes home from the hospital, after one day of recovery from a mastectomy, that doesn't make it okay!'" I tell her that Dr. Gioe only shrugged and said that it was the way things worked nowadays. I feel cranky. "Can you tell me when I can get more medicine?"

The assistant says she'll have to check with the nurse, and soon after that the nurse returns.

"Char said you were asking about medicine. Are you in pain?" she asks.

"I am!" I say to her.

"On a scale of one to ten, ten being the greatest pain, what is your number?" she asks me, a bit dubiously.

I give her my distressed look and answer, "Six."

She says she will look at my chart and see if I can have more medicine yet. When she leaves the room I say to my husband, "Boy, what if I said my pain was a nine, ten, or even eleven?"

"They would probably rush you to surgery," he says, slightly amused, "so it's probably good that you keep it to a lower number."

The nurse returns with a syringe and shoots it into my IV. I ask her what medicine it is and am told that it's morphine. I then ask her how often I will get it. She says I have to ask for it, but they can alternate giving me Norco every two hours followed by morphine the next two, and so on. So every two hours, I give my distressed look and my number six, and every two hours the medicine goes into my IV. With the medicine, I actually feel normal and without pain. I can sit up, eat, carry on conversations, and just be all around normal. In between it all, the catheter gets pulled out and the monitors come off.

When the time comes for the nurse's change of shift, I find that I'm actually looking forward to it. Every time my current nurse—who Richard and I have taken to calling Nurse Ratched—comes in to give me my morphine and Norco, I can sense her irritation. She doesn't seem to believe that I am actually in pain. I can tell by the way she quickly injects it into the IV, never making eye contact with me, and puckering her lips together to keep her judgmental thoughts inside. Heck, I don't even know if my pain *is* in fact a level six. All I know is that, as my mother would say, it is 2009, I just had my breasts removed, and I shouldn't have to feel *any* pain.

Bedtime finally comes and I get my final Norco shot followed by my morphine injection. My harsh, daytime nurse is finally leaving and I thank God that my body seems virtually pain-free. My husband lounges as far back as he can in the thinly cushioned, light-green recliner next to me. He tosses a white mesh blanket over his shoulders and reaches his hand towards me. I reach back and he bends forward and kisses my fingers.

"I love you, baby," he says sweetly.

I smile. "I love you too," I slur. "Thanks for staying the night with me."

~ ~ ~

"Oh my God, help me!"

It's 1:30 a.m. and I'm sitting straight up in bed, screaming. Richard jumps from his recliner and comes next to me.

"It's okay, we're in the hospital, you're dreaming," he says as he grabs my hand.

"Oh my God. NO, I'm not dreaming," I scream. "I need my medicine!"

The pain feels like someone has just chopped my breasts off. All I can feel is the raw, exposed tissue and me on no pain medication.

"Nurse!" Richard yells towards the doorway while he holds my hand.

The nighttime nurse comes running in and grabs my other hand. She is calm and smiles a no-need-to-panic kind of smile, which is so different from Nurse Ratched's scowl.

"Angela, on a scale of one to ten, what is your pain?"

I clench my teeth together, holding my husband's hand on one side and the nurse's hand on the other. I push out the number like I'm in labor: "Eight!"

The nurse leaves and returns quickly with both Norco and morphine at the same time. I believe she can tell my pain is more like an eleven.

"I thought I have to alternate these medications," I cry.

"For the most part, yes. But it is okay to give you both right now."

Had I known, I probably would have been asking for both at the same time. Within fifteen minutes I am back to a painless state. However, now my anxiety has increased as I'm thinking that I am going to die due to an overdose of Norco and morphine.

"Dear God," I say to Richard. "Do not forget to wake me every two hours." As I doze back to sleep, my last anxious murmur is, "I hope I wake up."

I've been so used to hospitals my whole life—psychiatric hospitals, medical teaching hospitals, conventional hospitals—mostly because I was visiting family members all the time. But now here I am having my first major operation in one of the biggest hospitals in our local area. ("Local" even though my husband and I traveled an hour and forty minutes to get here.) My one and only visitor is my dear old friend Cheryl, whom I've known from childhood. She comes the next morning, after my painful nighttime incident.

Cheryl and I have known each other since I was six years old. We were inseparable growing up and we would spend our summers tanning by her pool. July and August, in the late 1970s, consisted of baby oil for tanning by day, kick the can and hide-and-seek by night, and Pepsi and Doritos in between. My lifestyle has changed so much since then. Now I wear SPF50 and a garden hat, and I haven't had a soda in over ten years.

Cheryl comes in holding a beautiful wooden rose from the hospital gift shop. She hands it to me. "There's my oldest, bestest friend!" She then kisses my forehead. "I'm glad I got here before you had to head home," she continues.

It is now mid-afternoon, and I explain to her how I've been taking Norco and morphine every two hours throughout the night. I also tell her about Nurse Ratched and how having her back on shift makes me reluctant to ask for more medicine.

Cheryl takes care of this right away. She has been working in our little neighborly hospital near our hometown for over twenty years, where she is an assistant to an occupational therapist. She leaves the room and comes back momentarily, happily informing me that the nurse will be here with my medication. Nurse Ratched comes into the room and hands me my medicine in pill form. She seems less irritated and tells me she heard I had a rough night. Then she and Cheryl begin talking about their work in hospitals. The nurse leaves and tells me she will be back in a bit to go over my discharge papers.

My brother Ben calls me while I am in the hospital. I always love it that he comes through for me. The few other times I have ever been in the hospital, he was always the first to call. He called when I gave birth to my son, Matthew. He would have called when I gave birth to Adele, but I was home within ten hours of giving birth. When Ben finally caught up to me after the delivery, he earnestly asked, "Isn't that against the law? Them letting you leave so damn soon after giving birth?" Back then, I just held my belly and laughed.

Today when I talk with him I have to hold my chest while I laugh after he jokingly accuses me of being a faker. I continue to laugh with him and fade in and out of the conversation. When I am finally too groggy, I hand the phone over to Cheryl and happily listen to the drone of their talk.

I am just about to fall asleep again when the phone is ringing once more. This time it's my son.

"Hey Mom! How are you?"

My energy is low but I muster up enough to talk with him too. I mostly reassure him.

"Hi Sweetie! I'm okay, don't worry! I'll be home later! Hey, here's Cheryl!" I again pass the phone over to Cheryl and listen to her continue.

"Your mom is doing great, Matt!" Cheryl says, brushing my hair away from my sleepy eyes. On and on she comforts him for me.

In the meantime, Dr. Gioe shows up in full scrubs along with his three residents. Dr. Gioe looks insane today, though he still has his sexy demeanor. But there is something about him in the blue scrubs that make him look extremely intense. His wide eyes are bigger than usual and he has apparently just come from the operating room.

He holds my one hand with both of his.

"You look good there, lady!"

"Thanks, I feel pretty good." I smile back at him.

Another doctor reaches out her hand to introduce herself.

"Hi Angela, I'm Dr. Gioe's head intern, Dr. Harris."

I reach up with my IV hand because I want to keep holding Dr. Gioe's hand. I am even more drawn into his over-the-top and somewhat mad demeanor for some reason. But he lets go and shakes my husband's hand, telling him that I look good.

While Dr. Gioe and my husband talk, Dr. Harris begins to ask me questions. The other two interns are holding clipboards, and I hear them quietly talking about proactive surgeries, *BRCA1* positive patients, and genetic testing as if I can't hear them.

"Now Angela, how is it you came to be genetically tested for BRCA?" Dr. Harris asks.

When I start to answer, the two interns at the foot of my bed stop talking to one another and listen intently.

I share that I actually never knew there was such a test out there, going on to explain that a particular nurse, knowing of my family's cancer history, informed me that I qualified to be tested. I further add that when I had asked her why everyone didn't get tested, she had just shrugged and said that it was partly because it was too expensive. I go on to share what I know about these genetic tests and how the insurance companies handle them.

Since I find it very interesting that people in the medical community keep asking me about my genetic cancer test, I ask Dr. Harris why everyone keeps asking me how I came to be tested.

"It's because most people who get tested already have cancer," she begins, "and you don't. Obviously, this is a great thing."

With this pronouncement, I momentarily feel proud of my decision. I quickly change the conversation back to the issue of my next dose of pain medication.

One of the younger interns begins to tell me about Tylenol, but I ask if I can have what I've been having instead. I launch into my spiel about it being 2009 and how no one should have to feel pain, but she counters by telling me about the eighty-nine-year-old lady who just had a mastectomy and how that old woman is only taking Tylenol for her pain.

I feel a little bad, but not bad enough. "I still want my medicine before I leave today."

The intern looks over at Dr. Gioe, who gives her a nod. "Give her the medicine."

She coldly emphasizes to the nurse to bring me my last dose of morphine before I leave for the day. Then she instructs me to listen to the discharge information that the nurse is going to give me and to call the hospital if there are any problems, at which point they will connect me with the doctor on call.

I turn my attention away from her disapproval and praise Dr. Gioe for this whole journey he has been on with me.

"It has been my pleasure," he says, kissing my hand.

The nurse returns with my Norco and gives it to me. "I'll be coming by shortly with your discharge papers and prescriptions. You should pack up slowly and get ready to go."

"What time do you think I will be discharged?"

She looks at her watch. "As soon as I can get to all the paperwork, which will probably be after lunch."

Cheryl pats my leg. "I'll stay until you leave!" Then she takes charge by beginning to pack up for me. I thank her and close my eyes for my Norco catnap. Richard snoozes next to me in his familiar green recliner.

Cheryl has always been there for me. I remember when we were teenagers together and she got her first car, a sporty '78 Camaro.

I didn't have a car at the time, so she'd stop by to see me at my parents' home on Hollister Street. It was one of the best times of my life. I was seventeen and my family had a strong routine; dinners on Sundays, Frisbee in the summer, my dad bowling on Thursday night, and all of us watching *Little House on the Prairie* on Mondays and then *Dallas* on Friday nights together.

One particular Thursday evening, my dad needed a ride to his bowling match. He climbed into the passenger seat of Cheryl's Camaro while I sat in the middle, smack dab on the emergency brake. I swung my legs over Dad's bowling bag and laughed.

"I'm going to have to duck down if we see a cop!"

Cheryl opened her sun roof and started the car, while Phil Collins's "I Can Feel It in the Air Tonight" rang through the night.

Unbeknownst to me, in two years my father would be diagnosed with lung and brain cancer. He would suffer a steep uphill battle beginning in 1987, and die a mere ten months later.

I can feel it in my breath, my mind, and my heart today. I know that I have made the best decision ever—to have a full mastectomy. I want to have a strong routine and sense of family for my children, and I want to live long for them. I saw what cancer did to my family growing up, how it tore apart my dad's life and made the people around him turn to drugs, alcohol, and whatever else they could get their hands on. We needed to kill the pain of watching my dad dwindle down to mostly skin and bones. In his last few days of being alive on this earth, even the whites of his eyes had little black tumors on them. It happened so awfully and so quickly that the trauma from it still lives.

The nurse returns well after lunch—around three thirty in the afternoon—with my discharge papers. She reviews how I can't get the bandages wet, how often I should drain the tornado tubes, etc., but I mostly just want to see the prescriptions. When she hands them to me and tells me I can fill them tomorrow, I shake my head "no way" and ask my husband to go to the hospital's pharmacy and get them filled while Cheryl and I pack up. I want my medicine in my hands on the way home, especially after my "number eight" incident.

Richard takes the prescriptions and goes to the pharmacy. The nurse makes a real effort to smile at me and she even touches my arm. "I know you've been through a lot. Please call if you have any questions. We'll see you in three days to take off those bandages."

I get teary-eyed and think of my mom, dad, uncle, and grand-mothers. I touch her hand as I say, "Yes, my whole family has been through a lot."

When Richard returns from getting my prescriptions, a young man and Cheryl take me downstairs to exit the hospital in style—in a wheelchair. Richard leaves us at the rotating doors and goes to get the car. Cheryl kisses my forehead and says she'll be by this week to check on me. I thank her for coming and helping us today. I'm so thankful for long-term relationships like the one I share with Cheryl. I smile with a tear in my eye.

"I miss my mom and dad so much!"

"Me too!" says Cheryl, wiping a tear away.

As I get into the passenger side of the car, I tip the chair back into recliner mode for our hour-and-a-half journey home and I thank the young man who's already begun to take the wheelchair away. The young man then turns around and gives me a thumbs-up and a wink, just before taking the wheelchair back into the hospital.

Once we get on the highway, Richard reaches over and touches my hands.

"Are you doing okay?" he asks me.

I smile. "On a scale of one to ten, I'm a ten. God, am I happy to be going home!"

I close my eyes and fall asleep.

9

V for Victory, V for Visitors

When my dad was sick, at Syracuse's Upstate Medical Hospital, I had to drive the thruway in my Ford Pinto. I felt unsafe and insecure, not only because of driving on the highway but also because of the unknown and the fear of my dad's cancer. He had always been the breadwinner and had worked the night shift at Penn Yan Express as a dock loader for most of my later childhood. He was part of the Teamsters, so our family was financially secure and we had health and dental insurance, an abundance of roast beef dinners on Sundays, and loads of Christmas presents at holiday time.

My planned surgeries are about going back to a state of knowing, a mental space of security and safety like the one I enjoyed during the better days with my family. If I don't make the decision to move forward with preventative surgeries, I will always be on continual lookout, ready to fight a steep uphill battle like the ones that took five of my close family members.

My proactive surgeries are about leaving medical stress behind. Hell, life is stressful enough at times, so who needs the added worry? I made these decisions so I can let go of that fear and live my life with my family in the way that I want. Little do I know that I will have to be explaining this information to many of the visitors that come to see me over the next few weeks.

Our first stop before getting home is to pick up Adele. She is at my friend Jennifer's home, where she has been staying the past two days. We chose Jennifer because she is one of my oldest and dearest friends from childhood. We literally grew up next door to one another. Jennifer has two girls, one that is a year younger than Adele and one that is three years older.

Jennifer and her husband Korey are a healthy family, and we know they will be so kind to Adele. Their gracious help is in the form of a good family routine with family meals as well as driving the girls to school each day. I love it that I don't have to worry at all about Adele while going through such an event in my life. The more normal I can make it, the better.

When we pull into their driveway, it is dark and already almost 7 p.m. I tell Richard I want to go in with him.

"You sure?" he asks.

I say it will be good for me, so Richard walks around to my car door and holds his arm out for me to grasp as I shift my legs around and pull myself out of the car. I zip my coat up a little more to hide my tornado tubes. We walk in their back door and Jennifer greets me with a gentle hug.

"How are you my sister?"

"I'm okay, ready to go home."

As I am talking to Jennifer, I notice her eyes shift briefly towards my chest and then quickly back up to my eyes.

She yells to Korey who is in the living room.

"Korey, will you tell Adele her mom and dad are here to take her home?"

Korey walks out to the kitchen and shakes Richard's hand then hugs me.

"How are you?"

As I began to talk I again notice what I come to label the "Look, no chest!" look. I never judge or think badly of anyone who does it, I simply notice it. Whenever I talk about my mastectomy, people naturally give a quick glance to see if they can see my lack of breasts, and then return their eyes back to me and the conversation. I continue to notice it with every visitor over the next few weeks.

Adele comes running out to the kitchen with her school agenda, a shoe, a book bag, and her overnight sack.

"Hey, what took you guys so long? I thought you were coming to get me after school!"

I just smile at Jennifer and love it that my nine-year-old Adele has no idea about hospitals and operations or that I have tornado tubes holding my bodily fluids under my winter coat.

"We were goofing off!" I say to her.

Jennifer and Korey burst out a good laugh and any tension in the air immediately dissipates. I hug Jennifer again. "I love you. You're like my sister."

"I love you too. You are my sister." She gently pulls away and looks into my eyes. "Let me know when you can drink wine again. I'll come up and bring my mom so we can sit around and talk about everything."

"I can't wait!" I laugh, feeling so far-off from normal wine drinking and visiting. Then I need to hold my chest because it hurts to even chuckle a little bit. "Hopefully within a couple of weeks or so I will be able to do just that," I add.

When we pull into the driveway, I am glad to see my son's car. We are all now home together, just as I wanted. Matt greets us at the door and hugs me. My chest is already starting to hurt after having three hugs within the last thirty minutes. I begin to notice that the simplest tasks are difficult, like hanging up my coat. Just the act of lifting two pounds of clothing on a hanger makes my tight chest ache.

I take my first Oxycodone and smile the best smile I can conjure up for my family.

"I'm going to bed, everyone."

"Good idea, you get some rest!" Richard says as he kisses my forehead.

"I love you, Mom." Matt looks happy to see me get some rest.

"When you get better, maybe we can go to Splash Lagoon!" says Adele.

Her response makes me laugh so hard that I have to grab my chest. I am so far from Splash Lagoon material and so high on Oxycodone. My cry of laughter makes Adele give me a big hug. I compose myself the best I can, shuffle up the stairs, and crawl into bed without even brushing my teeth.

~ ~ ~

I wake at 1:30 a.m., sit straight up, and cry out, "Oh Jesus, help me."

I didn't set an alarm for my pain medication and now I'm experiencing the worst pain of my life. My whole chest feels like an open burn.

"Oh my God, get my medicine," I say to Richard, who is now sitting up in bed.

Richard grabs my pills and water from the night stand and hands them to me. Even though I'm crying, the pain is so unbearable that I actually start to laugh deliriously. I have clearly gone over some edge.

Richard rubs my arm. "Do you need to go to the hospital?"

"No!" I'm laughing and crying at the same time now.

"You sure?" he asks, confused.

"Yes, I'm sure! Just set the alarm, we can't let this happen again."

Richard empties my tornado tubes, which are full, and once we are on my new schedule, the tubes are only modestly full every few hours. I begin taking all the medication I can whenever the clock says it is time for more. In one instance, I'm unsure if I have even taken my medication or not, but I take a pill anyhow. Consequently, once I feel like the medication is becoming a routine pill blur, I begin writing down what time I took what medication. I'm certainly not going to let any of that pain stuff creep back into my life. It's almost 2010, and no one should have to have any pain, for God's sake!

My first visitor is my dear friend Maureen. When we were thirteen, we used to talk on the phone for literally hours. She even lived with me for a year during high school, shortly after her mom passed away from pancreatic cancer. Her first apartment was directly across from mine, just up the street from my parents' home. Though we rarely talk on the phone these days, we still never run out of things to talk about. She has the gift of gab, which I am sure is a prerequisite for being a hairstylist.

Maureen's salon is closed on Mondays, and she knows my friends from work are going to be coming in the afternoon after school is out. Therefore, she comes in the morning with her bin of hairstyling tools. Her plan is to make me look beautiful before they come.

She actually shows up a little on the early side while I am still in the bathtub.

"Perfect timing," I yell down to her. "You can help me get out of the tub."

She laughs and comes up the stairs. I am sitting in three inches of water so I don't get my bandages wet. I can tell by the look on her face that she is moved by my flat chest and tight bandages. She talks with me, pretending not to be moved or saddened and instead keeping a work-a-day voice so as to not show her feelings.

"Where should we wash your hair, you?" she asks me, her voice not betraying whatever sadness she might be feeling.

"Let's do it downstairs in the kitchen sink once I'm dressed. It hurts to bend backward, so bending forward might be better," I explain to her.

She cheerfully agrees.

"Whatever is best for you!"

Once at the kitchen sink, she uses all of her best things, washing my hair one time through with a tea tree shampoo, then a conditioning one, followed by a deep conditioner. She goes to work on me, primping and scrunching and fluffing virtually every strand of hair. Maureen is so sweet for taking care of me. While she primps, I kid her.

"I haven't had this kind of treatment since you were my 'Matron of Honor.'"

"How long ago was that?" She plugs in her curling irons and then laughs. "Remember how dark your mom got from the tanning booth? She was such a hoot. I miss her."

"Yeah! It was February '98, coming up on my twelfth anniversary." I smile. "Every other upstate New Yorker in the wedding photos had pale skin, especially mine with my off-the-shoulder dress." I hold my chest and laugh. "It was February in New York and Mom had to be tanned for those photos."

Maureen and I laugh and reminisce and by the time she is through it is nearly lunchtime.

I walk over to take more medicine.

"Want one?" I joke.

She laughs. "I would, but I'm not seventeen anymore."

When I look in the mirror, I see how good my hair looks, almost like I am going to a wedding. The ringlets are full and fabulous, all the way around my head, on top, and everywhere. My hair looks like a million bucks.

"Oh my goodness, it's beautiful. Thank you, Maureen!"

I want to wear the pajama outfit that my friends gave me, but they won't match well with my beautiful wedding hair. Regardless, I'm feeling new, fresh, and high on Oxycodone. Maureen hugs me and tells me to call if I need anything. She leaves me with her famous chocolate chip cookies.

When Richard comes in from the barn, I hold up my arms above my head like a big V.

"Your hair looks gorgeous," he says with a smile, and as he kisses me he rephrases his statement. "You look gorgeous."

I hold up my V again and say, "Victory!"

Feeling victorious, I continue to hold up my arms in the V stance throughout the day, shouting my Oxycodone slur: "Victory!"

This is my only form of exercise. Seeing how I have come from working out an hour a day doing yoga stretches, thirty minutes of aerobic exercise, and followed by ten minutes of weight training, holding up my arms in a V seems appropriate.

"What time are your friends coming this afternoon?" Richard asks me.

"Three o'clock," I say, and then realize I'll need to take my medication soon. I've decided to wear the robe, pajamas, and slippers my assistants had given me as gifts. Doris, my current assistant, got me the plush green robe with ivory stars on it. Sherry, my past assistant, got the matching green pajamas with an ivory paisley print. Gwen, a volunteer in my classroom, got me the ivory slippers. When they all arrive, I'll look put together, hair and all.

Patty backs in the driveway. Pam, Gwen, Doris, Jody, and Sherry get out and they all gather at the back of the vehicle, which is chock full of packages. When they come in through the front door, I hug each of them lightly. They are carrying gift bags and food.

Doris hugs me first. "There's more. We have to go back out to the car."

Patty hugs me next. "Oh my God! You look fabulous!"

"You look great!" Pam adds.

Gwen hugs me but doesn't say a word. She has a tear in her eye.

"How are you feeling?" Sherry asks.

Jody follows in behind carrying more gifts.

The gals pile the presents in the middle of the floor for me to open later. They put all the food on the kitchen table, and when Richard appears, Patty yells, "I made these chocolate chip cookies for you."

"I'll take one right now," Richard says with a smile. Doris right away begins explaining what the school is doing for me and my family during my recovery. She has that take charge attitude which, as my assistant, can be very annoying at times. However, my Oxycodone demeanor doesn't mind today.

"Okay, so let me explain what is going to happen here." She stands with her arms crossed and waits until we are all listening to her. "Twice a week, each grade level is going to bring you a big meal so you can have leftovers and you won't have to cook for the whole month of December. Matt and Val will be coming Thursday with more food."

I look at the quantity that is already on the table and can't imagine finishing all of it by Thursday. I'm overwhelmed by their kindness and can't believe how thoughtful my school is being to me. Everything from homemade bread, chili, cookies, tandoori chicken, rice, flat bread, and cake are in beautiful plastic dishes with bows on them.

"Each grade has coordinated, so there will be a lot of variety throughout the month," Patty chimes in.

I am speechless and wipe a tear from my eye. I can't believe how thoughtful my school is being to me. My friends each hug me again and I tell them to be sure that they thank everyone for me. Then I motion everyone to go in the living room where we can sit and visit.

We all sit around in the comfy furniture while Pam sits on the carpet with her legs crossed. I begin to recount my whole operation, telling them how one of my oldest friends came and did my hair, and how I have these tornado tubes underneath this robe. I give them a quick peek at the tubes. I don't show them everything but I feel I need to explain what is protruding from out of my robe.

My friends can tell I am getting tired and that I haven't even opened any of my gifts yet. Patty tells me not to worry, that I can open them later once I've rested. I thank them all for coming and once they leave I eat a cookie, take more pain relievers, and go to rest. Richard is coming out of the bedroom when I shuffle in. I hold my hands up again in the V shape and give a half-hearted, "Victory!"

This is what I do with every visitor that comes by; we sit in the living room and I process my operation (sharing all the gory details). Later, after the visitors leave, my family and I eat a wonderful meal. It is a therapeutic process and I wonder how people who rarely have visitors survive such a traumatic event.

～ ～ ～

When I wake up the next morning, nothing sounds good, foodwise. My stomach is nauseous from too much medication. The phone rings, and I notice from the caller ID that it is my sister, Chrissy.

"Hi, sweetie," she says to me when I pick up the phone.

"Hi, hon!" I respond, somewhat tiredly.

"I'm calling to let you know that I'm doing okay!"

I close my eyes and sigh disappointedly. She obviously doesn't remember that I just had a mastectomy.

"That's great, Chrissy! How are things at the new rehab?"

On and on she goes about how this time she is really done drinking. She starts to talk about her new roommate and how she is like a sister to her. Instead of saying what I'm actually thinking, I merely give her the best cheerleading I can muster.

"We're all rooting for you as usual," I say. I don't even bother reminding her of my mastectomy, I just contain my anger. "I have to go, hon."

"Okay, sis," she says happily. "When you do come up to visit me here, can you bring me some flip-flops for the shower?"

"I'll visit you as soon as I can, and I'll be sure to have them for you," I say.

As I hang up the phone, Richard comes in the kitchen.

"Who was that?"

"My sister," I disappointedly share. "Can you believe she didn't even mention my mastectomy? She totally forgot! Here I am with drainage tubes hanging out my chest . . ."

He rubs my shoulders. "Don't get all worked up. You know she has trouble loving herself."

I rest my head on Richard's shoulder. He always knows just what to say to make me feel better about any situation. As he gently rubs my back, I sigh and feel some of the anger towards my sister lifting.

Adele comes home and as she gets off the bus and enters the kitchen, Matt pulls in the driveway. I give Adele a big hug and ask her how school went, and when Matt comes in through the kitchen doorway he asks me how I am doing. I hold up my V. "Victorious!"

Adele smiles and runs upstairs. I can tell she is glad to be back to a somewhat normal home routine, with Mom spreading positive energy. As Richard goes into the living room to read the paper, I tell him I think I can make dinner. He asks me if I am sure, and again I hold up my V.

While I pull pots and pans out and reach in the back of the cupboard for something, I feel a pain in my chest. I lift my robe and I'm shocked to see blood soaking through all my bandages and gauze. My whole left side is drenched in blood and it has even gotten on my robe.

"Oh my God! Richard!" I yell.

Richard comes into the kitchen and when he sees my bandages he immediately says, "You should call the doctor's office before they close." He then scolds me and tells me to quit holding my arms up in the V or I will be victorious in heading back to the hospital.

I don't get a hold of my doctor, however I do have the nurse practitioner's personal phone number on hand. I call her and tell her all about how "victorious" I was feeling and that I had been holding my arms up, and how I felt I could even make dinner and get back to normal. She calmly laughs at my story and tells me to stop doing that and then asks when my next appointment is—which isn't until tomorrow—and says that if it gets any worse, I should carefully unwrap the bandages and see if the tube has come out. However, she seems pretty certain that I have just overdone it with my "victorious" stance.

"No more stretching!" she says. "At least not just yet. It's too early for that and it can make the scars stretch. You should just work on relaxing."

Her calm laugh as we end the call reassures me. I turn making dinner over to my son and my husband, and then yell to Adele to come sit with me in the living room so I can hear about her day at school.

Later in the evening, after Adele and Matt have gone to bed, my sister-in-law calls to check in on me. I tell her about my bloody event and laugh about doing too much, how I made my own breakfast and started to make dinner for everyone. As our conversation goes on, I can tell she is disappointed with my family when she asks, as though she can't believe it, "You had to make your own breakfast?"

I realize, at that very moment, that I deserve some waiting on as well. It makes people feel good to take care of me too, just as it makes me feel good to take care of others. For the next several days, I relish allowing my family to make my meals. And, really, they aren't making the meals per se. Rather, they are heating up the food that everyone has brought me. My school continually blesses me with food through the whole month of December.

The next day, Richard and I go back to Dr. Panilio's office to get my tubes taken out. Richard's been the one emptying the fluids from my tornado tubes these past few days. He tells me to sit back and enjoy the ride, which I know I will. I have just taken my medication, and I recline the seat and close my eyes. Richard turns on the radio.

I rest and think about my beautiful nine-year-old Adele and hope that someday they will have more alternatives for *BRCA1* positive patients. Maybe someday they can inject something into her to miraculously fix the mutated gene. This of course would be the futuristic Jetsons' way of taking care of a medical issue.

Even until this day, I still have my dad's wallet from when he passed away in 1988. In it he carried a folded up newspaper article which had information about the ultramodern CAT scans and MRIs being used to detect early cancers. I wondered if he thought about us kids, my brothers and sister, like I am thinking about Adele now, hoping for better technology to alleviate any unnecessary suffering.

When my dad died, I went on a health binge. I stopped smoking and started jogging. One night, however, I went out with some girl-friends, and while we were drinking in a bar, I began smoking again, and kept smoking for the next two and a half years. My binges were kind of like that. I did it all or nothing.

Once I had my son in 1990, I really began focusing on my health. My health binges turned into more of a basic healthy lifestyle, which occasionally included some potato chips and mozzarella sticks. I started doing aerobics. I really stopped smoking for good. When people ask me, "When did you quit smoking?" I can truthfully answer, "January 11, 1996."

I began eating greens like a rabbit and quit drinking soda too. I actually lost a bit of weight. Once I got my first teaching job in the fall of 1996, and then later my first public school teaching job in 1997, I had quite the health nut reputation. My mom called me her "flower child," which seems appropriate since I was born around the summer of love in the late sixties.

Anytime my mom came to my new home in the country, she always entered with a lit cigarette. I would shoo her back out the door. "Not in here, Mom. C'mon!" She'd step on it in the driveway and say, "Oh Jesus Christ, it's just a little smoke." Then she'd try to leave the cigarette butt in my driveway, which I would make her pick up and put it in her car ashtray. Every once in awhile one or two cigarette butts got by me, and I'd pick them up outside my home and roll my eyes and say aloud, "Thanks, Mom!"

My mom actually smoked just hours before she died in 2000. She had breast cancer, which had spread to her lymph nodes and liver. Every day, I called my mom from either the faculty break room at school or when I got home in the late afternoon from work. I remembered calling my mom from the break room at our school and telling her I was pregnant with my second child. I couldn't wait to tell her. The night before, I couldn't sleep and I bought a pregnancy test to use in the morning before I went to school. Instead, I got up at 3:00 a.m. and took the test, which came back positive. I never went back to sleep. I woke up Richard to tell him, told my nine-year-old son, Matt, before he went to school, then called my mom on my first break to tell her, and then blurted it out to all my friends at school. I was like two minutes pregnant and telling strangers about it. This was my type of personality. I never quite understood how women could wait until their second trimester to tell everyone that they were pregnant.

When my mom answered the phone, I cheerfully screeched, "Mom, I'm pregnant!"

She didn't scream out or get overly excited. Rather, she solemnly said, "Good, Ang! I'm happy for you!"

I asked her how she was feeling. She was probably taking prescription marijuana, prescription this, and prescription that. I just couldn't keep track of it all. I had a home, a husband, a son, a job, and now was pregnant again. I could take my mom for operations, call and check on her, but trying to control her medications, drinking, or smoking was something I simply gave up on doing.

My mom answered, "Oh, I'm okay. I'm just really tired today." This became her basic response to me, day in and day out.

One day when I called to check on her, she didn't answer her phone. I called my sister and said that we needed to go check on Mom. Her door was locked, so we crawled through her living room window and unlocked her apartment door. I yelled, "Mom! Mom!" Still there was no answer.

We went back to her bedroom, which reeked of stale smoke, and yelled, "Mom!"

Sure enough, there she was in bed.

"What?" she grunted.

"Jesus Christ, we thought you were dead!" my sister yelled.

My mom coughed, laughed a bit, and sat up in bed, asking my sister to pass her the cigarettes from the night stand. I scolded my mom and said we were going to get a key made for me because this was ridiculous, a pregnant woman climbing through the window to check on her mother.

My sister lit up a cigarette and smoked it with Mom. We all laughed and hugged, and I told them I had to get the heck out of there before the secondhand smoke killed me.

March 21, 2000
During work, I called my mom from the break room, only to find that her phone was busy. I called her again when I got home and the phone was

still busy. I was nauseous from morning sickness, so I told my husband I was going to take a nap. After I woke up I tried to call my mom again, and the phone was busy. I told Richard I was going downtown to check on Mom. It was dusk, around five thirty in the evening.

When I arrived, Mom's Oldsmobile and her other car were both in the driveway. Walking up the sidewalk, I noticed there were no lights on and my heart stopped. Thank God I had a key made to the apartment due to the last incident.

I opened her front door and gently closed it behind me. The smell of smoke was stale in the air; I could always tell my mom was home by the smell. It was always as if she went through spraying Aqua Net hairspray as an air freshener, but this moment that even smelled stale too. I yelled, "Mom!" There was no answer.

I yelled again, "Mom! Mom!" But nothing. I felt hopeless and squatted down against the door and yelled louder and angrier.

"Mom, answer me!"

There was no answer. I turned on the living room lights and then the kitchen lights and slowly headed towards her bedroom. When I entered the bedroom she was laying in the center of her bed, facing upward, eyes closed, sleeping. A small blanket covered her from her knees to her shoulders.

At the foot of the bed, I tapped her left lower leg.

"Mom, wake up!"

Her leg was frigid, and I knew she was dead.

I cried and quickly ran to the phone which was next to her and hung it up. I quickly run back into the living room and called my home. When Richard answered I cried, "Jesus Christ, Mom is dead!"

"Honey, you knew this was coming," he said calmly.

I didn't like his response. "Fuck you!" I yelled. Then I hung up and dialed 911. When they answered, I said, "My mom is dead!"

"How do you know?" they asked. "Do you want to try CPR? Where is your mom right now?"

I told them that she was lying in bed, that she had had cancer, and that it was too late for CPR.

They had me stay on the line with them and told me they were sending help. They kept asking me questions, "Are you sure you don't want to do CPR?"

I yelled and cried into the phone. "She's dead, I can tell. Her legs are cold."

I talked with them while sitting at the foot of Mom's bed, just looking at her. Her hair was perfectly sprayed and not one piece was out of place. Her eyebrows were done perfectly; black and drawn-in darker than any Joan Crawford look. Next to her on the nightstand was a pile of papers, bills, and more paperwork. On the other side of her was the phone which I had hung up. My mind raced. *Jesus she's been so stressed-out over that paperwork.* I ran with the thought. *Who was she trying to call? Me?* Perhaps she hadn't even been able to muster up the energy to call me or hang up the phone. I felt sick and told the dispatcher just that.

"Oh my God, my mom is dead, what happened?" I pleaded into the phone.

The dispatcher told me help was now at the apartment and that I should go and let them in.

I walked to Mom's front door where I found all of the neighbors I grew up next to, each one coming in to help me. They were all part of the volunteer fire department. Ray and Tracey were first on the scene. They were my family's lifelong neighbors. Ray's daughter-in-law, Lori, was with them. They all walked back to my mom's bedroom. Lori felt underneath Mom's arms and said she'd been gone for some time. Tracey, who I graduated with, took me by the elbow and walked me into the living room. He brought me some water and asked me if I wanted him to call his mother, who was my mom's best friend.

I said yes.

My mom and Marge were drinking, smoking, and parenting buddies for the past twelve years, ever since my dad died. However, they'd been a part of each others' lives for the last thirty years. Their family lived across the street from us. When Marge's husband Jack died, a few years before my dad did, Mom was there for her every day. And, when my dad died, Marge was there for her. Soon after, the drinking started heavily. They'd sit around, smoke, cough, and laugh, then head to the bar and drink some more.

Marge came right away and I asked if she wanted to go back into Mom's bedroom to say goodbye to her. She said she didn't want to go back there, instead staying right with me and talking about my pregnancy, the kids, and her grandkids while the paramedics did their thing in the bedroom. I could hear their walkie-talkies spiel off, "KD654, this is Yates County Fire Control, we have a woman by the name of Marlene Schmidt who is in need of the coroner . . ."

I talked with Marge and every few minutes I held my chest and cried. "Oh my God, my mom is dead."

It was like a nightmare, but real. Marge reached over and tapped my knee, as if to say, "I'm here for you." She didn't say a word, just tapped my knee with every cry.

The coroner came, and being how I lived in a small town, I knew him too. He talked with the paramedics and I could hear them explain how I was pregnant and I was the one who found her. He then came over and gave me a hug. He got real close to me and held my face.

"Angela, I'm going to have someone drive you home." He looked at Marge and gave her a wink.

I tried to explain that I was fine to drive, but he shook his head. "I'm going to have someone take you home." He then told me I couldn't stay for the next part and I had to leave. He told me they were going to put Mom in a bag and take her to the hospital. He explained that he knew she had had cancer, but an autopsy would be necessary to determine the actual cause of her death. Just then, the local funeral home owner walked into Mom's apartment, touched base with the paramedics, and then told me to give him a call the following day.

I gathered my purse and my Mom's blanket from the couch. I threw it over my shoulders, and Marge and I walked arm in arm to her car. When I got in the car, I propped my head up and felt more nauseous than ever. I only lived five minutes away and Marge talked the entire time. "Ang, if there is anything you need from me, please let me know. Our family is here for you."

We pulled in the driveway and Richard walked out to greet us. I buried my head in his chest and cried. Marge touched his shoulder and repeated the same message to him. She told us she would call the following day.

∾ ∾ ∾

December 14, 2009

When Richard and I arrive at Robert Packer Hospital we take the elevator right up to the fourth floor to Dr. Panilio's office. We have gotten to know the hospital and all the floors like the back of our hand; even signing in and dealing with our insurance cards is now a snap. Right away, the receptionist knows us, saying, "Oh, hi Angela. We're going to take you right in, we had a cancellation."

Richard comes with me, and as instructed, I undress from the waist up. Dr. Panilio comes in shortly after the nurse leaves, shaking my husband's hand and greeting him with his Filipino accent. Then he turns to me.

"Let's have a look." He opens my gown and sees the blood covered bandages. "What happened here?"

I start to laugh and tell him how I held my arms up above my head too much, shouting, "Victory!"

He nods knowingly. "Yes, that'll do it," then tells me he is going to remove these bandages and get fresh ones. He unwraps the tight gauze and has me lie back on the table, telling me he is also going to remove the tubes.

"Are you ready?" he asks, right before beginning the process.

I'm obviously worried about the pain. "Is this going to hurt?"

"Like a quick bee sting," he says. "Easy, fast." Then he adds, "On the count of three I'm going to pull these out, are you ready?"

I squint my eyes and grind my teeth. "Okay!"

He counts "one" and then just as fast as he can he rips them both out at once.

I hold my chest. "Oh my God! I thought you said on three!" It feels like he tore out the tubes from my lungs.

He laughs and pats my knee.

"You're okay!"

Richard looks in pain from just watching, and I'm in disbelief as I hold my chest.

"Oh my God! Are we done, is that it?"

"That's it!"

Dr. Panilio instructs that I can get back to normal and begin bathing in a few days. He adds that the nurse will be coming in to bandage me back up. He explains how he will see me in two weeks, and that we will start adding fluid to the tissue extenders. We will do this every week until I am at the bra size I want to be. Once I am at my desired size, we will schedule the reconstructive surgeries for removing the tissue extenders, inserting the saline implants, and then make a decision about the nipple reconstruction as well.

I feel so much gratitude for not having cancer, and so fortunate to be proactive with my health. On the way home, I talk with Richard about my dad and his unfortunate experiences before the doctors ever figured out he had cancer. He lost his job, began acting odd, sleeping on the couch and breaking out in soaking sweats, and then of course there was his stay at the psychiatric hospital that lasted nearly twelve weeks. He did receive a few weekend passes to come home, however.

By that time, Dad had gained some weight in the stomach area and his polo shirts were too tight. He had slippers on and shuffled around the kitchen, pacing back and forth with a lit cigarette in his hand. He definitely looked like a psychiatric patient. I kept a positive attitude and pretended nothing was different.

"C'mon, Dad, why don't you sit down?"

He'd take a drag of his cigarette and numbly mutter, "I don't want to sit down." He kept shuffling and pacing, doing the Thorazine shuffle.

His last full day on earth was August 5, 1988. I was at my apartment sitting on the porch steps, smoking a cigarette. My brother Ben pulled up in Dad's brown Ford Granada, rolled down the window, and said, "Hey Ang, you better come up to the house, Dad doesn't look too good."

I quickly put out my cigarette on the sidewalk and said I'd be right there. I went into the apartment and told my boyfriend, Al, that we needed to go see my dad. When I got to our family home, Dad was laying wearily on his hospital bed in the living room. I sat on the edge of the bed.

"Dad, you okay?"

He painfully grumbled, "Uh huh."

I looked up at my brother and mom standing in the living room.

"We should take him to the hospital."

I knew Dad said he never wanted to go back to another hospital again and that he wanted to die at home, but my mom was high on medication, my brother Ben came to get me because he was worried, and my fifteen- and sixteen-year-old brother and sister were already bewildered. Besides, I just thought the hospital was a place where we could safely be together and make the necessary decisions. We could let the professionals do what they needed to do to help Dad. I defended this decision by adding, "Maybe they can give him some medications, and we'll be home before we know it."

Mom acted angry.

"Well, are you going to take him?"

"Let's call Ray. He'll bring an ambulance," I responded confidently.

So we called our next door neighbor Ray, fire chief for our local volunteer fire department, instead of 911. Right as the ambulance pulled up outside our house, Uncle John walked in and asked what was going on.

Once we explained our plan, he gathered up his cigarettes and my brother and sister, and we all headed to Ithaca Hospital where my dad's oncologist, Dr. Ulrich, was based. We followed the ambulance in our two family cars. There wasn't a lot of talk, just numbness and disbelief.

Once in the emergency room, we all gathered around my dad's bed. When Dr. Ulrich came in, I pulled her aside.

"Is he going to make it?"

She then said, "No." She shook her head and touched my arm.

"He's not going to make it through the night, honey."

I became more shocked and didn't reply at all. I thought, *How can this be happening? He hasn't been sick very long. This can't be it. That's not how it goes. I know he's been fighting an uphill battle, but people recover and die at a later time, not a mere ten months from diagnosis. This isn't later. What's happening?*

Dr. Ulrich circled around the bed with all of us and put her hand on my dad's shoulder.

"Stan, do you know where you are?"

My dad painfully mumbled, "The hospital."

"Stan, tell me who these people are."

My dad looked up and I could see that little black tumors, almost wart-like, had formed on the whites of his eyes. He limply pointed to Mom.

"That's my wife."

He looked towards my younger brother and sister.

"That's Anthony and Chrissy."

He pointed to me.

"That's Poopaa."

He looked over to my brother Ben and reached out.

"That's my boy."

We all started to cry, knowing that my dad adopted Ben as a toddler, when he married my mom in 1967, something we never found out until Ben was twelve; Dad raised him, loving him as his own.

Dad was too tired to continue. Dr. Ulrich gently tapped his skinny arm. "Stan, we are going to get you a comfortable room where your family can stay with you."

Dad, in a loose fetal position, shook his head yes, letting her know he understood what she was stating.

By the time we got in the private hospital room, it was late afternoon. We took turns leaving to go smoke, eat, use the bathroom, or whatever else we could do to avoid what was happening. Around dusk, Al and I went down to the first floor and sat outside the hospital. I sat on the sidewalk with my back against the brick wall, lit up a cigarette, exhaled, and cried. I felt ashamed for smoking, knowing Dad was dying of lung and brain cancer. I didn't want to feel any of this. I just wanted to stuff it down with nicotine.

When we went back up to Dad's room, we were walking down the long hallway and about halfway to Dad's room we could hear him painfully breathing. This breathing continued throughout the rest of the night. Later, a young priest came to read my dad his last rights, but before doing so he tried connecting with the family by offering some offhanded jokes that weren't funny. I was pissed off, angrier than ever, and wanted to go smoke some more, but refrained from doing so. After the priest left there were a few times when Dad was staring into the air and painfully uttering, "Dad, Dad!"

I wondered if Grandpa was coming from Heaven to help him leave the Earth. Once 6:00 a.m. arrived, I told my family that Dr. Ulrich was wrong because Dad made it through the night. Mom directed Ben and me to take our younger brother and sister home to get some rest, shower up, and come right back. Mom and Uncle John would stay with Dad.

So, we left the hospital. Ben and Al sat in the front, and Ben drove. I sat in the back in between Anthony and Chrissy. They were sleeping in a curled-up position all the way home. It was a solemn forty-five-minute drive. Ben dropped me and Al off at our apartment and said he would be back to pick me up at eleven so we could head back over to the hospital.

However, I was woken up at 9:00 a.m. by my uncle pounding on my side door. I opened the door and looked out, noticing Mom was in the passenger seat of the car. "Ang, your dad is gone. We're going home to rest. Your mom says to come up later." I furrowed my eyebrows, still in disbelief. *I'm supposed to go back to the hospital and hug him more*, I thought.

He died on the morning of August 6, and we buried him on August 8, 1988. I remember watching the news that evening in my parents' living room. People all over the world were celebrating because it was 8/8/88, and there wouldn't be another date like it again until 9/9/99. I stared into the television set as the news story went back and forth from Australia to the USA, covering all of the people with horns and party hats. I muttered, "I just buried my dad."

In the car and on our way home from my appointment, I explain to Richard about how the people partying on TV actually taught me that life does go on. It was as though they visited me on that auspicious day to say, "You must choose to live." I decided to fully live life again, and live a life that was a spirited one. I tell Richard how I eventually quit smoking. My dad died at forty-two, and I wasn't going to die at an early age. I never want my children to see little black tumors on my eyes or hear me breathing painfully. I sure as heck don't want them to ever use the word "cancer" and "mom" in the same sentence. When Richard and I pull in our driveway, he kisses my hand and tells me how proud he is of all my decisions, especially my decision to marry him.

10

Bereavement and Resolutions

I just want to be normal again. I begin my prayer, "Please let me get back to taking my life for granted, as I had before. Okay, not really! I don't want to take my life for granted, but I do want to get back to living my life like I did prior to this operation."

I am thrilled that I can now hang clothes up without pain. I feel an incredible sense of gratitude for the simple things, like walking and bathing. I want to get back to my yoga body so badly. I actually get down into plank position and try to slowly lower myself to a hover but I cannot do it without pain in my chest. My anxiety feels high because in just a few short weeks I will be having my hysterectomy, followed by reconstructive surgery. I am, however, determined to get back to a somewhat normal life.

It doesn't take long for the universe to answer my prayers.

The phone rings one day, and when I answer I hear an unfamiliar voice.

"Hi, Angela, it's Dee, Penny's cousin. How are you?"

"I'm good," I tell her. "How are you?"

"I'm good as well," she replies. "You're probably wondering why I'm calling you. Well, I'm on the emotional health committee for Our Town Rocks. Our committee has been talking about you and we were hoping you can teach yoga to our community. Of course, we'll pay you for it, and we'll do all the advertising. Is there any chance you could meet me and Gail to discuss the details tomorrow, say around three o'clock, at the Youth Center?"

"Of course, that would be great! See you then!" I hang up the phone and put up my arms above in a V and feel health run through my body.

I show up to the interview wearing my yoga pants, however I throw on a large zip up hoodie to cover my extremely flat chest. I certainly want this job—heck, I asked the universe for it. In the back of my mind, there is a small fear that if the Our Town Rocks committee finds out I just had an operation, they might think of it as a liability issue and cancel the thing altogether. However, I know my good attitude and vibrant demeanor will win over my fear today.

Gail and Dee are at the conference table, and right away I recognize Gail as we were once in a Sunday meditation group together. We all connect and make some small talk about the holidays. I have come into the interview fresh and with no medication since I want to appear as healthy and vibrant as I can. Although I am in some pain, I know I can fake it until at least the interview is over. I explain to them what I need financially to take on the class and share that I can make a flyer and that they can use it to advertise. Gail and Dee are very gracious. They tell me they have money to buy yoga mats for all the participants, and my first book, *Seeking Balance in an Unbalanced World*, about health, wellness, and balance for everyone. They are certain they can fill the room to guarantee me a good salary for my once a week yoga training for the community.

"How soon can we get started?" Dee finally asks.

I pull out my calendar and say, "How about March 21?"

I know, in the back of my mind, that I have my hysterectomy scheduled for February 3, and I'm scheduled to have my saline implants inserted a couple weeks later. I won't be doing my nipple reconstruction until spring break, which is in April. This will allow me to do a six week class beginning March 21, and I can have the option of cancelling one class in April and bumping it ahead one week due to my nipple reconstructive surgery.

So we decide that the yoga class will begin on the first day of spring. Gail and Dee are excited and we all exchange email addresses and shake hands. When I get into my car to go home, I open my pill bottle and take a Tramadol. I think, *I can do this! I want my yoga self back*.

Driving home, I think about how auspicious it is that I prayed for this and the actual day that I am going to begin *Stretch into Spring* is on the anniversary of my mother's death. It is so hard to believe she has been gone nearly ten years already. I remember the day of her funeral like it was yesterday. I was just six weeks pregnant, and being the oldest girl in my family, the burden of the funeral was put on me.

My two brothers came to my home to meet the priest, Father Peter. During our meeting, we told Father Peter that we invited our sister to come but she was struggling with my mom's death. We further explained rather bluntly, that she was probably drinking instead. Father Peter wanted to do a good job for us at the funeral, so he came right to my home to inquire about my mom's life.

He began with a reminder that a funeral is a time to celebrate a person's life. My heart was having a hard time celebrating. I was still having morning sickness, but with my brothers here, we got in a few laughs about Mom, and many sad stories too.

We told Father Peter about Mom growing up in Flint, Michigan. We shared how she ended up here in Dundee because she married our father. We told him how, after Dad died, she was never the same, and how her alcoholism had spiraled downward. She simply never recovered. We offered him the one memorable example of the downward spiral.

I looked at Ben. "Do you remember when the bartender called us from the Waneta Inn Bar and said they'd taken Mom's keys?"

Ben crossed his arms in front of his chest, sat back in his seat, and nodded a yes. I continued filling in the story for Father Peter.

"Yeah, Ben and I walked into the bar and Mom's upper body was basically sprawled across the countertop. When she saw us, she looked up and slurred, 'Hey you guys! I didn't know you two were coming here!' Ben reached out to the bartender and the keys were discreetly handed over. We ordered her a soda, lied to her that there was vodka in it, and Ben and I played two games of pool at the pool table while Mom passed out across the bar again." I wiped a tear from my face. "Then we brought her home and tucked her into bed."

Father Peter stayed with us until late afternoon and then said he had enough information to prepare his eulogy. He sat back in his chair and looked at his notepad. Then he took a deep breath and looked at the three of us and added, "It sounds more like your mom died of a broken heart than of cancer."

We all hugged him, and he touched my arm and looked in my eyes.

"You took good care of your mom. You should be proud of that."

I was grateful that we chose Father Peter to present at the Catholic funeral.

We had a private viewing of my mom at our local funeral home the day before the church funeral. It was a small gathering; my godmother and her husband, Mom's best friend Marge, my two brothers and their spouses, my sister and her boyfriend, my mom's brother Frank, my Aunt Jean, and Mom's two sisters, Eva and Deb, all came from far away. I went to my mom's apartment the day before and chose a purple sweater and black stirrup pants. I also chose some blank onyx earrings, a necklace, ring, and bracelet for her.

In the casket, Mom's hand held my grandpa's rosary. We all entered the viewing room, and for the second time in my life I saw my brother Ben cry. The other time was when we had all gathered around my dad in the emergency room on his last day on Earth. I hugged Ben, and he wiped a tear away.

"You did good, Ang," he said to me.

Everyone was teary-eyed, and there was a solemn feeling in the air. Then we began our Polish family talk. Within minutes of our conversations starting, our folding chairs had been rearranged into an oval shape. Uncle Frank and Aunt Jean began to laugh about a time when my mom was young, and soon everyone was laughing and talking with their hands flinging this way and that.

This continued into the evening and lasted well over two hours, all of it full of laughing and chatting about Mom. Every once in awhile, I looked up in the front of the room and saw Mom in her casket, and felt sick in my gut. But I always returned a smile to my Uncle Frank's boisterous laugh.

Baird, the funeral director, came in and whispered to me that we needed to say our final good-byes to Mom as she was going to be sent for cremation. Our calling hours were private and we scheduled them to be from 7 to 9 p.m. However, when I looked at my watch, it was now after nine thirty. Our time together as a family had been beautiful, and it flew by. I allowed everyone else to go to the casket first, opting to stay in the back of the room and watch all the others kneel at the casket, saying their last good-byes.

After my sister Chrissy had finished her prayer by the casket, I knelt down by Mom's side and placed my hand over hers, which held the rosary. Her hand was cold. I closed my eyes and paused. I felt at ease knowing her heart was not broken anymore. I felt a certainty that her spirit was now with my dad's. I took a deep breath and whispered, "I love you, Mom."

The next day, Father Peter met us at the church forty-five minutes prior to the church service. Ben and Anthony pulled in at the same time. When they got out of their cars they asked me, "Where's Chrissy?"

I just shook my head in disbelief.

"I'm not sure."

Father Peter consoled us. "Well, we are early. There's time."

We headed into the church, and Father Peter pointed for us to sit in the front row with our spouses, followed by my Uncle Frank, Aunt Jean, Aunt Eva, and Aunt Deb. He showed us how the flowers on the first three pews were for family and close friends. We moved into to our seats, and the 1:00 p.m. time came. The church was now filled with neighbors, my colleagues and bosses from work, my mom's friends, everyone. Everyone, that is, except my sister. When one fifteen came and there still was no sign of Chrissy, Father Peter finally began the service.

"Let us pray!" he began. "Before we get started, let us pray for Marlene's daughter, Christine. She is having a difficult time with her mother's passing." He discussed how she was the youngest, the baby of the family. "Let us have a moment of silence for her."

I bowed my head, mostly pissed off at my sister for not being present.

Father Peter then began talking about Mom's other children. He started with Ben, talking about his life in Kentucky, and followed with Anthony and how he came all the way from Saratoga Springs with his wife.

As he began to talk about me, the church doors suddenly flew open. In came my sister with her longtime boyfriend. My cousin was with them as well. They were all wearing jeans, and I could tell by my sister's sway that she was drunk. In her drunken demeanor, she took notice of people on her way down the center aisle, continually acknowledging this person or that one by saying, "Hey, how are ya?"

I was mortified. I motioned for her to come to the front, but she shook her head no and blurted out, as she squeezed through people in a pew a couple back from ours, "I'm fine back here."

Father Peter calmly took charge and interrupted his eulogy.

"Welcome!" he said, and then continued. "And then there is Angela, who is Marlene's oldest daughter. She had Marlene's oldest grandson and is soon to have another child."

Then my sister interrupted again, shouting, "Hey, I'm her daughter too!"

Father Peter stopped again and replied, "Yes, I know, we mentioned you first and prayed for you."

I could not believe there was now a conversation going on between Father Peter and my sister in the middle of Mom's service. *Are you frickin' kidding me?* I thought. I was completely embarrassed and humiliated.

"You don't need to pray for me," my sister slurred and then looked down at her hands.

Thankfully, she kept her head down and the rest of her drunken words to herself. I actually thought she had momentarily passed out in the pew.

As Father Peter continued, I felt sick and shameful.

"At least your boss won't question why you put in for eight bereavement days," Richard whispered to me.

I smiled at him and almost burst out a tense laugh. I had to immediately look down because I didn't want anyone to see me laugh at my mom's funeral. Richard smiled and grabbed my hand. I was instantly taken back to a feeling of gratitude and thanked God he still loved me despite my sister's behavior.

It is hard to believe this particular incident happened nearly ten years ago. I realize how much I have already gone through emotionally, having had to bury both my parents before the age of thirty-two. Now that I am forty-one, I stand strong in my emotional decisions to have two preventative surgeries. I want to be here for my children, as a solid rock. I want to live a long, long time, to the point where I can shout out senile things when I am ninety-two and have my great-grandchildren laugh at my confused and silly mental state. I am proud of these personal decisions I have made.

～ ～ ～

Dee calls me two days after advertising *Stretch into Spring* and informs me that the class is already full. There's even a waiting list. She excitedly shares that we should already be thinking about doing a summer session. The books and yoga mats have been ordered and there is nothing more I need to do other than show up on March 21 with my yoga music. It is the end of December. I would be heading back to work in mid-January for a short two and a half weeks and then take off some more time to heal after my hysterectomy. I'd also take time off to have the surgery for my implants.

On New Year's Eve, I pour myself a glass of wine and sit down in the recliner to write out my 2010 goals. It is a relaxing holiday. My son has headed up to Montreal, Canada, to bring in the New Year, and Adele has taken a nap because she wants to get up and stay up until midnight. I make a broiled salmon dinner with brown rice and asparagus, and I have a small bottle of champagne to bring in the New Year with Richard (even though I know he won't drink it). At least he'll toast with me by holding up his Columbian coffee. I have been so proud of Richard's choice to not drink alcohol. He has been alcohol free since 1980 and I love that he feels the strength of a healthy lifestyle. It is important to us as a couple.

My goals include getting my body back to the most flexible healthy state I can ever be in, along with my writing aspirations and the regular old resolutions that don't always get fulfilled. I star the goal about my body and even write down some prerequisite goals to get there, such as teaching the wellness class this spring and perhaps even teaching yoga to some friends at school. I take another sip of wine, close my journal, hold it to my belly, take a deep yoga breath, and think, *It's going to be a great year—the best one yet!*

11

Changing, Inside and Out

February 3, 2010

I can hardly believe it is already time for my hysterectomy. It has been exactly eight weeks since my mastectomy, and I go through the same type of routine. Adele stays with my friend Jennifer, Matt takes care of our pets, and Richard takes me to the hospital. Everything is prepared, and I am ready to go.

Once at the hospital, I notice the facilities are a little older than Robert Packer Hospital where I had my mastectomy. However, they are clean and simple and I am mostly satisfied with Dr. White.

"Would you like a little something to calm you down?" she asks me when she comes to my bedside.

"I do," I say to her as I wipe a tear from my eye. "Do you ever take medication?" I ask this because I really want to get off all of my medications but I am weary of throwing them away because I might need them when I get home.

She wipes my hair from my face, nods, and warmly smiles at me.

I smile and feel normal, or as normal as I can feel lying naked on a gurney.

Dr. White then tells me, "We have a good team here today, and we're going to take good care of you!" She looks up at my husband and gives him a wink. He is at the foot of my bed holding my cold toes. "I'll come and find you and let you know how she's doing," Dr. White says to him.

Richard kisses me and reassures me that he will see me soon. Before I know it, I am again being wheeled down a cold hallway, on a gurney, high on Versed.

When I come to after the operation, a nurse tells me my husband will be meeting me back in my room. They wheel me there, and I find Richard sitting in a straight back chair. He stands up and out of their way as they move me from the gurney to my hospital bed. He kisses my head and asks me how I feel. I touch my lower abdomen and say, "Empty," then add, "hungry."

The nurse, who's listening to our conversation, says she will be bringing me food soon. She then tells Richard that I can have water for now.

Richard gives me a cup of ice water from the little plastic pink pitcher. I joke about it, knowing we already have one from my last operation.

"Now we'll have matching pitchers at home."

He kisses my head again. "That didn't take long."

I have lost my sense of time and notice it is very gray outside.

"How long was I in there?" I ask him.

"I'm not sure how long the actual surgery took but from the time they did the surgery through recovery to now, it was only about two hours. You look good, though."

I am sure I look frazzled as heck, though.

"I have to go pee. Can you tell the nurse?"

When the nurse comes in, she reminds me that I have a catheter in. I touch myself down there, and sure enough there is a tube.

"Well, can you get it out?"

"I'll be right back and then I will help you to the bathroom," she responds.

I look at Richard.

"Did I have a catheter when I had my other operation? I don't remember the catheter feeling like this." It feels very uncomfortable, and the more I focus on it, the more I want it gone. I quickly remember that I did have a catheter during my other mastectomy operation. "I can't believe I forgot about the whole catheter thing."

When the nurse returns she brings a nurse intern. "This is Liza. She is studying to be a nurse. Do you mind if she is here while I remove your catheter?"

I am uncomfortable and irritated and respond with a blunt, "No, I don't mind. Please get it out."

The nurse pulls the covers off of me and touches the tube. I can feel it pull inside me and I put my hand down near the nurse's hand.

She moves my hand to the side and says, "Don't touch." Then she shifts her attention back to her nursing student. "The urethral catheter just gets a quick tug," she says as she yanks it out, "and there. We're all done."

I look at the ceiling, feeling more uncomfortable than ever, and add, "Dear Lord!"

The nurse taps my leg. "You're okay. Come on now, let's go to the bathroom."

They each hold an arm of mine and help me to the bathroom. I tug along the IV and its rollers for the big pee event. Once on the toilet, I sigh and feel relieved that it still feels normal peeing without my cervix, uterus, ovaries, and whatever else they took out.

They shuffle me and my IV back. I crawl back into bed, and soon after my food comes. I try to eat but my stomach is bloated and full and I have pain, therefore it is time to again ask for more pain medication. I am, however, determined that once I am out of this hospital, no pain medication will be taken. But, while I am here, I will take what I can take. Mostly because that is what my mom would do, and because it is 2010 and sure as heck no one should be in any pain in 2010.

I tell Richard he doesn't need to stay with me and that I'll be okay. I don't want him to have to sleep in a hard chair again. He takes my advice, and I take my mom's advice from Heaven, "Just take the medication. It's there for you." And so I do, and sleep well.

∽ ∽ ∽

The next day Richard comes to get me and I tell him I can't leave yet because they want me to have a bowel movement. When the nurse comes in, I ask if they can give me some medication to have a bowel movement. She says she'll check with the doctor. Later, Dr. White comes to see me and tells the nurse that I can be discharged, however she looks back at me and says if I have any problems when I get home, and I don't have a bowel movement, I should give her a call. I hold her hand and thank her for all she has done.

Soon thereafter, a nurse comes with a wheelchair and tells me I am being discharged. She gives me two prescriptions: Darvacette for severe pain and Tramadol for daily pain. I take them and make sure Richard stops on the way home to get them filled.

"Don't you already have Tramadol?" he asks me.

"It'll be backup," I say, and he shakes his head but still gets them filled at the pharmacy while I sit with my hands on my lower belly. On the way home, I open the Darvacette and take it with some ginger ale.

When we get home, the kids greet me and I crawl into the recliner and ask Richard for the heating pad. I feel even more bloated than ever. I still haven't had a bowel movement and I'm becoming worried, especially since my whole lower abdomen aches.

I put a call into Dr. White the next day, and later she returns my call and tells me all about Miralax and Sennocides and Ducolax. She informs me that Ducolax will even make me go to the bathroom within the hour. When I get off the phone with her I ask Richard to go to the pharmacy to get some. He asks which one to get. I bark at him and tell him one of every kind. He should get me everything, I need to go to the bathroom.

I can't believe how much I hurt. I moan and groan, holding my belly and whimpering, "Jesus, help me."

When Richard returns, I take one of everything he bought, and sure enough within the hour I go. Thank God—I never knew that constipation and gassiness would be a major side effect of this operation. I never realized that pain medications slowed everything down, especially your digestive system. I learn it all the hard way, literally.

Within days, I start feeling better during the daytime. Nighttime is a whole other ball game. I begin waking anywhere from an hour and a half to every forty-five minutes with hot flashes. I had heard about hot flashes with menopause, however being young and fertile, and as someone who gets her period literally every twenty-eight days, I'd mercilessly judge anyone who would say they had hot flashes. My mind would say, *Big deal; a hot flash? Try having tumors grow out your eyes, and you can't make it to the bathroom because you're nothing but skin and bones because cancer has eaten away at your whole body. Hot flashes, really?*

However, my kind reply I always used to give was, "I heard black cohosh tea works great for hot flashes." Then I would quickly change the subject, because really who wants to talk about boring hot flashes, anyway?

Of course this is my karma. My judgments come back to haunt me, or worse, give me extreme hot flashes. No one tells me that once your female organs are ripped from your body, and you are whipped into menopause, that menopause hits you like a truckload of bricks. I can handle the hot flashes during the day. I can make myself appear like I am glistening by dabbing sweat with a tissue, drinking water, and covering up my uncomfortable hot flash with a positive attitude. And, because I am so busy taking care of two classrooms during the day, I barely have time to notice. Seeing how I do need to care for so many children, sleep is unbelievably necessary, however it just isn't happening. This is how Ambien comes into my life and becomes my new best friend.

Oh my God, I love it. I hear people talk bad about its addictive qualities. Once I told a woman that I was taking Ambien. Her face expressed concern and she warned me to "watch out." She then shared that she had an addiction for three years with it.

I tell her I am not going to be on it long. Seriously though, I have to weigh my circumstances. I always know when a hot flash is coming. They begin in the center of my bones and work outward until my bones are like heat logs, radiating like an oven through my muscles, and into every jiggly part of my body. But between getting no sleep or some sleep, well, it is a no brainer.

My general family doctor even has a problem with me being on it, telling me about black cohosh tea. I think, *Black cohosh tea, my butt.*

My pharmacist tells me about melatonin and how we need it to sleep, how our bodies make it, and how, as we get older, we don't make it as much. I think, *I'm forty-one years old, my body is not old.* Then, when she tells me you have to take it for sixty days before it truly gets into your system, I think, *Sixty days, my butt. I'll be dead by then. I'm so frickin' tired, just give me my Ambien and leave me alone, I'm not hurting anyone.*

When I discuss the Ambien issue with Dr. White, she tells me I can be on it the rest of my life; she doesn't care, especially if the quality of my life improves. She writes me a double script for it so I can have two pills if I want to, or just have some for backup. I side with Dr. White's advice and begin taking the Ambien at eight o'clock every night. If I do get a hot flash in the night, I simply say to myself, using my Ambien mind, "Oh, you're just having a hot flash, now go back to sleep." And I do.

Dr. White also tells me to continue taking Neurontin three times per day. These will help with the hot flashes as well. This becomes my daily regimen, and for the most part it works. However, fatigue from too much medication creeps in slowly but surely.

I have also been going every week to add more fluid to my tissue extenders. How they do it is actually quite interesting. There is a magnetic port just under the skin so that the needle knows exactly where to poke. The nurse practitioner has been doing my saline injections and she has started out by giving me only 25–50 ml of fluid. I so want my breast size to be ready by mid-February that on one occasion I tell her I can handle more fluid at one time. She inserts 90 ml and it hurts me to breathe that evening because I have stretched out my skin too much at once. My body is saying to me, *Hey, take it easy. Easy does it.*

Nonetheless, I am bound and determined to get "the girls" up to the size I want them to be, and to do so by mid-February. I don't have a lot of days left for sick-time, and I don't want to deviate from my plan, regardless of what my body is saying to me.

My husband takes me again to this operation as well, and we are definitely old pros by now, knowing the exact route we want to take to the hospital and how long it will take to arrive. Once we get to Robert Packer Hospital, we check in and they tell me this is a quick in-and-out procedure. They refer to it as outpatient surgery. I'll be home by dinner.

Again, I am put under anesthesia, and when I come to I feel nauseous. I am again wrapped tightly in bandages. They are around a special bra that I am instructed to keep on until my next visit. I am given an antibiotic and told that this is to be taken in case my body rejects the foreign objects now inside of me. I even got a ten year warranty card for "the girls." I am happy to have the tissue extenders out of me. They had felt as hard as rocks and I am told my implants will feel very soft and real.

I make my follow up appointment with Dr. White and Dr. Panilio on the same day so I can kill two birds with one stone. I will head all the way to Dr. Panilio's office in Pennsylvania, eat lunch, and then backtrack home, stopping for my appointment at Dr. White's office. This time, my godmother will go with me. It will be nice to have someone to chitchat with on the way. My godmother drives. My chest is feeling uncomfortably tight in the special bra and I tell her I can't wait to get these bandages off.

When we got to the hospital, I check in with Dr. Panilio's receptionist.

"Angela, he'll be right with you. You can have a seat in the waiting area."

My godmother and I sit directly next to one another so we can whisper and not let others hear what we are talking about. She leans in towards me.

"So this is it, you'll be all done after today, right?"

"I need to think about what I am going to do with my nipples," I whisper back.

She shrugs. "What are you thinking?"

"I have three options," I begin. "I can do nothing; I can have a medical tattoo, kind of like a 3D tattoo of a nipple; or I can have a skin graft, where they take skin from my groin area and make that into a nipple."

My godmother nods, leans in again, and whispers, "Go for the real nipple thing."

"The skin graft choice?"

She nods yes. "You've come this far, why not do it right? You're young. You should have a real nipple."

I agree with her. "You're right. You know, I'm going to ask when I can get that done. It's a whole other operation, but it would be my absolute last surgery."

Just then the nurse comes out and says, "Angela?"

I stand up and my godmother hits my arm.

"Go for the real thing."

"Yeah, I will," I say confidently.

When the doctor comes in, I ask him almost immediately about the nipple reconstruction. He tells me I can have nipple surgery sometime in April, after I heal a bit. I share about my precious sick days and how I'm hoping I won't have to take off anymore time from work. I really want the nipple reconstruction to be done during my spring break vacation. He assures me that he will work with me on whatever date I choose. I ask him if I will also need a tattoo to make the skin darker for the areola. He again tells me where he will be taking the skin from, and that the skin is already a shade darker down there. Therefore, when it is grafted into my chest it will be a tad darker, and I won't need a tattoo at all. He explains that it will even get a bit darker over time. He'll use that skin to make a protruded nipple as well. He explains how he will have to overextend the protrusion because in time it can lose some of its protrusion.

At this point, I trust him explicitly, and after he looks over my new implants he tells me I am good to go and that he will see me in April. When I leave, I make the appointment with the receptionist for my April nipple reconstruction. I walk out to meet my godmother in the waiting area and smile and tell her, "We're off to my next doctor appointment."

All of my decisions are solidified. We head over to Dr. White's office for my follow-up from my hysterectomy. I have noticed all through my earlier lunch that the center of my chest itches like crazy. I try not to be too obvious, but I can't help digging right in the center of my chest. I ask Dr. White if she can look at it. I apologize that I didn't have Dr. Panilio look at it and share that I just came from his office. However, I tell her how I got all caught up in preparing for the next operation: my nipple reconstruction.

Dr. White seems interested, and as I unbutton my shirt, she nods in approval.

"Wow! They look good, Angela." She wheels her little stool a bit closer to look where I have been scratching. She says, "It looks like a yeast infection."

I scratch it some more and say, "I didn't know you could get a yeast infection up here."

Dr. White tells me to stop at the drug store and pick up some over-the-counter medication to put on it. Then she has me lie back to take a peek at my vaginal area. She tells me, "You look good down here, too." Then she helps me sit up and asks if I have any questions.

I tell her about wanting to stay on the Ambien for now and ask about how to get off the Neurontin. She explains that if I am going off of Neurontin, I should do it gradually.

"I kind of have another question, but it's a lengthy one."

Dr White dries her hands and sits down.

"I always have time. What's your question?"

"Okay, so women who are BRCA1 positive have a forty-four percent chance of getting ovarian cancer. And Dr. Murphy had explained to me that, with BRCA positive patients, they found out that if they just removed the patient's ovaries that the tumors still formed in the fallopian tubes."

Dr. White nods as she follows my train of thought.

"So doctors started removing the fallopian tubes. However then they noticed that tumors formed in the uterus, so they decided it was best to remove the uterus and then the cervix as well."

Dr. White nods again.

"Well, what about the vagina? Wouldn't cancer form in the vagina as well? And if so, what the heck do they do about that, remove your vagina? They can't remove your vagina, can they?"

Dr. White reassures me by saying, "I see where you are going with this. Don't worry. You should see all the amazing things they can do now.

If there ever was cancer in the vagina, they can skin graft and create a new one. But you don't have to worry. You have done everything in your power to be proactive. You are good to go. No worries!"

I feel so happy with her response. I love it that both of my doctors tell me I am good to go. I feel good and give her a hug and tell her I will see her at my next follow-up. When I get out to the waiting room, I cheerfully say to my godmother, "We're good to go."

That evening, I pour myself a glass of red wine and begin making my Italian penne pasta dish. Richard comes in through the kitchen door carrying his lunch pail from his day's work. He comes over to the counter, kisses me, and, looking down at the fresh garlic, tells me, "Mmm, I can tell that it's going to be a good evening."

I kiss him back. "Hey, I've got something to tell you."

"What?" he says as he pops a tomato in his mouth.

I explain how my godmother took me to both doctor appointments today, and he interrupts.

"Oh yeah! How did it go?"

I am surprised that he forgot I had two doctor appointments today. I think he is just happy to be back at work and that he doesn't have to take me to any more hospitals.

"Well, I made up my mind. I'm going to have the full nipple reconstruction," I smile and finish with, "in April."

He looks surprised. "Wow! That's right around the corner."

"I know, but then I'll be all done with surgeries. I can heal before summer and be back in a bathing suit." Then I throw my arms up like an excited teenage girl at seeing a boy she likes. "And then I'll be back to normal."

I find it interesting that "back to normal," at the age of forty-one, equates to the same feelings of teenage puppy love.

He kisses me again. "Whatever you want. I support you."

I chop the vegetables and think to myself how lucky I am to have all this timed just perfect, and how I won't have to take off any extra time from work. *This is perfect. Thank you God!* I think.

ᕲ ᕲ ᕲ

As the spring break vacation gets closer, I am walking down the hallway after dismissal time at school one day and two veteran teachers are sitting on a cement ledge that overlooks our school courtyard. I stop to say hi. Julie is discussing her upcoming trip to Florida and how she is excited to stay in her new timeshare. Terry says she is heading down to DC to stay with some relatives. Then she turns to me. "You doing anything special over spring break?"

I smile and quietly lean in. "I'm having surgery."

Julie's face drops.

"Oh Angela, not again. Is everything okay?"

I assure them that this is a good thing, that this is the last part of my reconstructive surgery, and I am actually quite excited about it because then I can truly focus on my healing. Julie still looks sad, so I give her a hug and say, "Really, this is a good thing." Then Terry stands up to give me a hug too.

The day of the surgery comes around quickly. It is a quick in-and-out type of operation. The nurse doesn't even refer to it as surgery, rather saying "a procedure." Here I am again at Robert Packer Hospital. Some of the nurses who have gotten to know my face even come over to say hello to me. One asks, "Where's your husband?"

I tell her he is out in the waiting room catching up on some reading. She informs me that Dr. Panilio will be right with me.

Dr. Panilio comes through the curtained area where I am sitting on my gurney. He opens my hospital gown and says, "Let's have a look here."

He then takes out a purple marker from his pocket and sketches on my chest where the nipples will be put. As he does this he shares, "I used to measure precisely when I first started out, and now I just do it by eye; it looks better that way."

He finishes his last marking and then has me lie back on the gurney. He makes purple ovals in my groin area, one on each side where my underwear would be if I had any on. This is where he is going to take the skin to form my areola and nipple. He finishes up and asks, "Okay, we're all set. Do you need anything?"

He means medication, and this is kind of like happy hour, so I say, "Yeah! That would take the edge off."

A nurse comes right away, starts my IV, and soon I am just a little high on Versed, which has become my new surgical friend.

When I come to, the nurse brings me some water and says I can eat soon. She tells me she is going to get my husband and comes back with my discharge instructions. I look down at my chest, which again is wrapped tightly in gauze and bandages. I peek down at my groin, which hurts worse than my chest area. Each area is bandaged up and I have a pair of disposable hospital underpants on. I picture myself under anesthesia and them lifting me to put those disposable underpants on. I wonder how many disposal underpants the hospital goes through in a day.

The nurse comes back in and brings me toast, apple juice, a pain pill, and my husband. Gratitude comes over me and temporarily sends the pain away. I start to cry tears of joy for being finished with all my surgeries. Everything in life is just perfect.

12

Caring for the Girls

Today is the day they are going to take off all the bandages and show me my new nipples. It is like an unveiling and I can't wait to see them. I have extreme pain in my groin area when I walk, therefore I am moving around very slowly. White pus has formed on the incision in the left groin area. Each time I use the bathroom, I pull the gauze off and then dab some peroxide in that area with a cotton ball. I want to show Dr. Panilio my groin incision first. When he comes in the room he asks, as always, "How is it going?"

"Pretty good up here," I say as I touch my bandaged chest, "but I think I have an infection down here."

"I'll fix you right up," he reassures me. He looks at both incisions in my groin area. "Yes, a slight infection. We'll give you something for that. Let's look at what we got here," and he unwraps my chest bandages.

I look up at the ceiling until he has them completely unwrapped. He is saying, "Oh yes, these look good, very good."

Despite his positive words, I am still scared. But I look down anyhow. When I do see my new nipples, I shout so loud that I'm sure the patient in the small room next to me can hear.

"Oh my God, they look awful!"

The nipples are swollen, crusty, and bloody. Black stitches are poking out of the protruded part and all the way around the areola.

Dr. Panilio laughs.

"What do you mean 'oh no'? These look good!"

I laugh too. "Really? These look good?"

"Yes! Wonderful!" He pulls out one little black stitch. "All of these little stitches will just fall out when you shower," he says, holding it up.

I look down and still can't believe how many stitches there are; moreover, that they will just fall out on their own. I assumed that things were going to be perfect right away. I wish someone had told me about how things really look horrible in the beginning, how it takes time for things to heal and to really look good. I again have to find this out for myself.

"Let me show you how to take care of your new breasts." Dr. Panilio reaches into his cupboard and pulls out what appear to be breastfeeding pads. "This is really simple, but you have to do it twice a day until you come back here in two weeks."

He first takes a pair of small scissors and cuts two small incisions right in the center of the nursing pad. He holds it up, showing me the cross cut in the pad. Next he squeezes antibacterial ointment on the center of the pad and then softly places it over the center of my new nipple. It feels quite soothing. He then hands me the other pad and asks me to try it on my other nipple.

When we are finished with my lesson, he gives me a front-snapping bra. "You're good to go. Again, do this two times: once in the morning, once in the evening. I'll see you back here in two weeks."

He writes me a prescription for Tramadol, which is now stockpiled in my medicine cabinet, and then another prescription for an antibiotic for the slight infection in my groin area. I make my last follow-up appointment and then drive home. However, I stop at the pharmacy first to fill my prescriptions and buy all my necessary supplies for my new daily nipple regimen, something I'm dreading having to do.

I walk into the pharmacy and head right to the Band-Aid aisle. There is a middle-aged woman already in the aisle and she has no hair and a blue western bandana tied around her head. She has an oxygen pack on her waist; it is in a kind of leather black carry bag. It looks light to me, but it appears heavy for her to carry. She is so pale and thin that I can't help but notice her bony hand and wrist; then I look at her face. She doesn't have eyelashes. She looks at me and smiles, and I smile back. I think how incredible it is to be suffering so deeply on so many levels—physically, emotionally, socially—and still have a smile to give. I can only guess that she has some form of cancer. She grabs a large box of Band-Aids and then excuses herself as she walks past me down to the cashier.

Alone in the long aisle, I began to nonchalantly put things in my carry basket. I toss in more white tape, gauze, antibiotic ointment, and then I grab the same brand of Band-Aids that the woman had just picked off the shelf. I hold them in both of my hands and read the package, ALL PURPOSE PROTECTION.

I just stare at the large box and begin to cry. I miss my mom. I miss my dad. I miss my uncle. I miss my tiny breasts. I miss not being able to do a yoga backbend and raise one leg in the air. I miss my husband not being with me today. The feelings come hard and I can barely breathe. I look up at the ceiling and cry, then back at the Band-Aids and all of a sudden I start to laugh and cry simultaneously. A young man turns down the aisle, sees me crying, turns around and goes down another aisle, which makes me laugh even more. I grab a tissue from my coat pocket and gently wipe my tears and say out loud, "Just how much gauze can one person buy in a year?"

I laugh at my own joke and fill up the carry basket with everything else I need. When I get in the car, I take in a deep breath and feel better. I feel grateful that I don't have cancer and I don't have to carry around an oxygen tank. I feel happy with my jiggly stomach and the little bit of extra weight I have put on. When I start the car, the radio is playing Journey's "Don't Stop Believing." I crank it up and sing at the top of my voice the whole way home.

~ ~ ~

The next day is school, and while in the bathtub in the morning, I begin to pick at the stitches and pull out what ones I can. I become obsessed with getting the stitches out, as well as peeling away the dry crusty skin that is all around the nipple. My new nipples look nasty, and my whole goal now is to get back to the attractive state that I used to be in.

I look at the clock and notice I am late. I still have to apply the ointment pad, so I dry off quickly and begin my new regimen. I start by cutting the nursing pad, making a small cross in the center of it, and squeeze a ton of ointment on it before putting it over my nipple. Then I put on my bra, followed by another nursing pad so the ointment doesn't get my bra oily. I sure as heck don't want grease spots on my shirt. I already feel so exposed at work; the more inconspicuous, the better.

Now I am really late, and I yell down to Richard, "Hey Fish, can you throw me together an egg sandwich for the road, I gotta go. This is taking more time than I thought."

"What's taking more time?" Richard yells back.

"My frickin' nipple thing," I shout back and laugh. "The nipple frickin' ointment crap."

Richard is never frazzled in the morning. He's always calm. He doesn't work for anyone else, though, and he doesn't have children waiting at the door when he gets to work. He yells up the stairs, "An egg sandwich to go, come on now," letting me know that I'm really late.

He rushes alongside of me and carries my breakfast to my front seat. As I am backing out the driveway, I roll down the window and yell, "I'll do better tomorrow."

He puts his hands together in prayer and nods to me in the Namaste stance, the one I always do at the end of each yoga class with all of my yoga students. I have taught my students that Namaste means, "The light within me salutes the light within you." I have instructed them to silently offer a "Namaste" to the people they see in the grocery stores and other places, especially the distressed ones. I laugh and blow him a kiss from my window. If my yoga students could only see me now, all frazzled and busily hurrying myself off to work!

On the way to my job, I look down at my chest and feel like I look inordinately big. The extra nursing pads add more stuffing to my now larger breasts. I laugh out loud, "Larger breasts . . . this is now my problem!"

Due to how long my new nipple regimen is taking me, I now start to get everything ready the night before. I cut the two nursing pads beforehand and put out two regular ones to catch any seepage. I placed the ointment on the sink just to save time looking for it in the morning. I also begin bathing at night so I can obsessively pick away at the dry crusty skin and pull out the stitches that are supposed to miraculously "wash away."

By the time two weeks have gone by, my new nipples look perfect. They aren't quite symmetrical; however, my original ones weren't either. When I look in the mirror, I notice the eye isn't drawn to the scars anymore. Rather, my eyes see round, full breasts, a lot rounder than my real ones were. My old breasts were tiny 36Bs. They were droopy from breast feeding two children, but they served me well. I really don't miss them anymore, and I love my new 36Cs and perky nipples. I can't wait to show Richard. I had been hiding the unsightly plastic surgery until I was completely healed.

One night, when the kids go to bed, I put on my sexy silk camisole and matching loose panties. I am happy it covers my groin scars. I crawl into bed with Richard and whisper, "Want to see my new breasts?"

He turns and squeezes me.

"I'd *love* to," he says, and starts to kiss them. "Oh my, they're beautiful." He kisses them again and finishes with "You're beautiful."

I never tell him I can't feel the kiss on my breast, but I lie back, smile happily, and feel good about my new body and life.

The next day, I put on my new Victoria's Secret wireless bra and go to see Dr. Panilio for my follow-up visit. Underwire bras are now a thing of the past for me, as wireless bras help "the girls" last longer. When Dr. Panilio comes in he gives his usual, "How are you doing?"

I tell him I am good and happy, which makes him chuckle. He says he likes happy patients and then adds, "Okay, let's have a look." He then opens up my gown to take a look at how my new nipples are coming along. "They're beautiful. I can tell you've been doing a great job." He then touches my left nipple. "We can adjust this if it bothers you that it is pointing downward."

I throw my hands up in the air.

"Oh no, I'm good. No more surgeries."

He then puts both of his hands on his knees.

"We are finished here, then. I don't need to see you anymore, unless there is a problem."

"A problem?" I ask.

"If they ever leak or anything and we have to put in a new one, we will just go in from the side so as not to obstruct the new nipple," he says, pointing to the part of the scar on the side of my chest.

I ask a few last questions.

"Can I sleep on my belly? I've been sleeping on my side. I'm wondering if that would hurt them."

He taps my knee. "Sleep on them. You can do whatever you want now."

I thank him for the whole journey and jokingly add, "I hope I don't have to see you again."

Before he leaves the room he turns to me. "These look good."

I stand up to get dressed and look in the mirror and whisper to myself, "You look good, Angela."

13

The Lows of the High

I am very excited that I am getting to where I want to be, physically, emotionally, and spiritually. So, early one morning, I open up my journal and look at it. Underneath my goal of getting my yoga body back, I add one more item: get off the medications. At this point I am still using Tramadol throughout the day for pain, taking Ambien to sleep, and Neurontin three times per day for my hot flashes. I feel fatigued, and this has become my typical state of being.

I don't have an actual plan for how I am going to get off the medication, especially since my doctors tell me to take them as needed. One of my turning points comes when it is late after school one day. I have stayed late to work on my progress reports and checklists. I have just taken my second Neurontin of the day when my friend Heywood comes to see me.

"Hey Fish! Why are you here so late?"

I am exhausted, and I'm certain that my daily fatigue is caused by the Ambien I take each night before bedtime. I take it because my hot flashes have been so intense that I am waking up every forty-five minutes. My doctor had initially told me to take Neurontin for my hot flashes. "It tricks the brain into feeling pain differently," she had said. "Take the Ambien to get a good's night sleep; you might wake up from a hot flash, but you will go back to sleep immediately. Hopefully you won't even wake up during these night sweats." She really convinced me by adding, "Getting good sleep improves the quality of your life. So, if you have to be on it for your entire life, then I am perfectly fine with that."

Here is this wonderful doctor that I admire and look to for advice. She is perfectly fine with me being on these medications for my entire life. She is perfectly fine even though Ambien is a highly addictive medication. I see the need for quality sleep. I see the need for improving my life. Therefore, I start taking my Neurontin and Ambien each evening, just before bedtime. At first, I sleep better than ever. I never loved sleep so much. Then I take my Neurontin in the morning before school. I take a second Neurontin during the day. And, when the kids are dismissed, I usually take a Tramadol if I'm in pain. Later, I drive home completely exhausted and start this medication routine all over again.

So my turning point comes when I am conversing with Heywood. I notice my words running together slightly and I try to act like it didn't happen. Heywood is like a brother to me so he doesn't act like it didn't happen; rather, he mimics what I just said.

"My progress reports aren't finished," I try to say, however, it comes out in a completely worn out, done-in, exhausted manner.

"My progresh reports aren't finish."

Heywood tries to mimic me.

"My progresh report aren't finish," he says. "What the heck kind of medications are you taking?"

I haven't had to confront anyone about this until now. I've only been calling the doctor and leaving a message that I need a refill, and boom, it happens. All I have to do then is go pick it up at the drugstore. I had switched some of my loopier medications to a pharmacy a few minutes further away, that way I wouldn't have to confront my personal pharmacist who is a friend of mine. Heck, I even began having my husband or son pick up the drugs for me.

"What do you mean?" I ask Heywood, pretending not to know what he's referencing.

"Just kiddin' ya, Fish! My report cards aren't finished either. That's why I'm still here." As he leaves, he holds up his hand with a peace sign. "See ya, Fish!"

It is now getting dark outside. I look out the window and wonder, *Am I taking too much medication? I am doing a fine job teaching during the day. I'm only taking my Neurontin during the teaching day and limiting my Tramadol use until well after the students are dismissed. Yes, it is spread out throughout the day, but it still feels like a lot.* My last and best thought that solidifies my turning point is, *I am completely frickin' exhausted and I hate how I feel.* I have now officially confronted this issue, and that is thera-peutic enough for this day.

Beforehand, when I asked my doctor's about taking the medications at work, both of them assured me that it was fine. I am only taking my sleeping medication at bedtime and my Neurontin in the morning, afternoon, and just before bed. The Tramadol is the kicker—that loopy type of medication. I typically only take it once or twice a day. It is a "take every four to six hours" medication.

I notice Tramadol also helps me in coping with my assistant, an older, abrasive woman working with my little pre-K students. My boss tells me they put this new assistant in my classroom so I could "help her to be positive." He shares that they want her gruff attitude to be transformed into a more positive one, like mine.

For the most part, I think I do a pretty good job of doing what my boss has asked me to do. However, at some point I realize that you can lead a horse to water, but you can't make it drink. So, knowing that I can't change her, I have come to some sort of mediocre tolerance with her behavior.

It has become second nature to me, when she scolds a little one: "Caleb, get your hands down off the wall."

I calmly turn to my class in the hallway and say, "Brian, I like the way your hands are down by your side." I try to teach her positive rein-forcement by then adding, "Oh, and look: Caleb, good job on putting your hands down now."

Or when she snaps at the little ones during lunchtime, saying, "Ryan, close your mouth when you're chewing, this isn't a farm," I counter with, "Look at Brianna, she is doing a good job with her lunch manners." I always add a teaching piece: "Ryan, great job, you're now chewing with your mouth closed."

This type of interaction continues throughout my hours at work. It is stressful and tiring, a part of my work for the past six years, day in and day out. This is the component of my job that has started to consume me. This task alone exhausts me, not to mention me giving my best positive attitude towards my little three- and four-year-old students. I need my classroom to be a reflection of my philosophy. Snapping orders and scolding children definitely doesn't sit well in my heart. Therefore, I can't wait to take a Tramadol when I am in a wee bit of pain.

I begin to also notice that I take a Tramadol when I feel annoyed. Rather than a pain medication, it has become more of a "get rid of annoyances" type of medication. One day, right after school, I turn on the big interactive whiteboard. "Doris, I've got to show you an episode of *The View*," I say excitedly.

Doris is cutting out items from tagboard for an art project. She is irritated and throws up one hand.

"Oh, I hate *The View*. Everyone is always fighting and angry at each other."

I tell her that this isn't about *The View*, but rather an interview they did with a woman newscaster from Fox News. I explain how she had the same preventative operation as I did; however, this lady didn't even test positive for a mutated gene. Some of her family members had died of cancer, and so she chose to get tested but tested negative. She was then put back into the ranks of people who faced the usual odds of ever getting cancer. I thought her story was extraordinary because she trusted her body more than any medical test. She felt that she would always wonder if she was going to get cancer because of her family's history. Her surgery was a little different than mine, in that she had the nipple sparing mastectomy. Nonetheless, I connected with this extraordinary woman.

I find the episode just before we are leaving for the day and show Doris the quick five minute interview. I am so impressed by this woman that I excitedly toss my hands up.

"Doris, can you believe how courageous she is? She didn't even test positive like I did!"

Doris keeps cutting the tagboard, and looking down, she bitterly says, "I don't understand why women are having these operations when they don't even have cancer."

This time, my jaw just drops at her nastiness. She looks over at me, and I can tell by her sour, angry face that she is spitefully pleased with my disappointment.

"That's just my opinion," she says.

I shut down the computer and I'm done for the day. At this point, I feel done with Doris too. I can hardly believe that, after everything I have gone through, this is the type of support I am getting, and from someone who was supposed to be my assistant, no less. I grab my purse and leave for the day. Halfway home, I take a Tramadol.

When I get home in the evening, I open up to my husband about everything, including the two episodes at work. I tell him about Heywood noticing my words running together. I tell him about Doris and her cold judgments. I open up about how I completely and thoroughly frickin' hate the job of teaching an antagonistic, spiteful, and unsupportive assistant how to be positive. I tell him I hate my Tramadol use too. It's as if I am in a Catholic confession booth again.

The one thing I have always loved so very deeply about my husband is that I can tell him every feeling I am ever having and I know he always loves me. He loves me even knowing my worst feelings. He has a way of focusing on the wisdom in virtually any situation. He calmly points out, "Maybe notice that she is a suffering individual that has never healed."

I cry and hug him.

"You're right."

Richard adds, as he holds me closer, "Begin each day like you are meeting her for the first time ever."

I laugh into his shoulder and again say, "You're right."

Then he holds my shoulders and pulls away to look at me in my eyes.

"Try taking the Tramadol when you're only in pain, not just annoyed."

I wipe away a tear and agree.

I keep taking the Neurontin for hot flashes three times a day, but I stop taking the Tramadol altogether and just deal with my annoyances by being direct, like telling Doris that I need her to assist me, not go against my educational philosophy.

I make the decision to speak directly, to stop taking the medications that make me feel loopy, and I add more yoga, relaxation, and meditation in my life. The combination of all these things greatly improves my strength. It is a remarkable recovery to be in control of the parts of my life that will help me be the healthy, strong woman I want to be.

When I talk with the doctor about going off of the sleep medication altogether, she recommends that I should go off it gradually. I then begin my regimen of taking the sleep medication every other night. It then goes to only a few times a week, and finally to no Ambien at all.

I don't want to be like my mom, who carried a heavy purse with eight or more pill bottles for every ailment. She had the type of pills from, "My nerves are shot" Valium, to "My throat hurts" amoxicillin, to "My back hurts" two Valiums and one codeine. Therefore, I make the decision to wean off the Neurontin as well.

I go to visit my local pharmacist friend, Tracey. I now openly discuss my use of Ambien and Neurontin, and she points me towards the beautiful natural supplements in her store. She shows me how I can use Melatonin for sleep and black cohosh for hot flashes and night sweats. I talk with my doctor as well, who also believes it will be best to gradually go off the Neurontin. Therefore, I only take one Neurontin at night and drink black cohosh tea during the day. Within a few weeks, I am off the Neurontin altogether.

I have come to an acceptance about taking Evista. Evista was originally developed as an invasive breast cancer medication. But scientists discovered that women who took Evista didn't lose any bone mass, which is a common issue for women who have their female organs removed. This is especially worrisome for someone who is as young as I am. I certainly don't want to get osteoporosis, like my mom.

Therefore, taking Evista is a win-win situation. First, it will be helpful in preventing invasive breast cancer. Most people think that just because you have had a mastectomy that you can never get breast cancer. However, doctors can never get all the breast tissue you have. A mastectomy only lowers the chances of getting cancer to just below five percent, which is still terrific odds, especially from where I started at the over eighty percent mark.

For that reason, I make the decision to keep taking Evista after my hysterectomy. Evista will be the medication I take for the rest of my life. The one side effect that Evista has is blood clotting. So, I also choose to take a baby aspirin daily.

I have now basically gone off all medications. I keep the things that give me energy. I have limited my medications to Evista and a baby aspirin, and then start a heavy-duty vitamin regimen. I begin taking a calcium supplement along with a separate vitamin D supplement. I start taking vitamin B, C, and E, and after dinner another calcium/vitamin D combined supplement. At bedtime I take fish oil, garlic, more C, and another baby aspirin.

I think, *My God, I feel good.*

14

The New Woman

When I was in my teens, I did all sorts of crazy things, thinking I was indestructible. I recall my friend Denise and I, at around thirteen, stopped at the top of a Ferris wheel, and how we rocked the seat acting like we were going to flip it over, whooping it up, yelling "woo-hoo!" and naïve enough not to know that we might actually be able to do it. When we got off the ride we were laughing. "We're still alive," we yelled gleefully.

Somewhere along the line, I realized that indestructible didn't really exist. Permanency was a façade, everything was fleeting. I had watched enough of the news by the time I was in my twenties to know that people *did* die on roller coasters and on other amusement rides. More importantly I had seen my own parents die, my dad passing away when I was only twenty years old and my mom when I was thirty-one. Therefore, I learned to sit nicely on Ferris wheels, and when I had my own children I told them to hold on tight and to be extra careful.

I had worried about death, never wanting anyone close to me to go before their time. Then I learned about the BRCA gene. Up until then, I had always thought that lifestyle was basically the only determinant of cancer. And although I knew lifestyle was critically important, I now faced the truth: genetics could be even more powerful in determining someone's death. I had seen people with "good" genes smoke into their eighties and drink whiskey into old age too. I had seen my own family members die very young.

After all of my surgeries, and all the emotional issues I have gone through, I can see that something drastic has happened to my psyche. I have become a new woman. It's as though I have brought back my thirteen-year-old spirit to hangout permanently with my

After teaching my yoga class for six weeks in the spring and practicing a lot of meditation, I decide to live like there is no tomorrow. I begin doing things I would have only done as a naïve girl. This time it is even more powerful because I am not naïve, I know better. Granted, I am not trying to rock myself off of a Ferris wheel, but I refuse to let any fear control my life. I decide to be more present. I decide to live, period!

One day, soon after April break, I enter the teacher's lounge at school. Some of my colleagues are asking one another, "What did you do over spring break?"

"I finished my fourth operation," I share. At the end of my story, Heywood walks in.

"Hey Heywood," I say as he walks through the door, "you missed my 'I just finished my fourth operation' story."

He holds his hand up to his mouth and opens and shuts his fingers together several times really fast as he jokes, "I know, I know, you just had forty million operations so you wouldn't have to work again."

I laugh out loud, knowing Heywood only teases people he likes, and with that joke I know he loves me very much. Then his face gets kind of serious.

"Want to go whitewater rafting down the Black River?" he asks.

At first I think he is joking, but then he starts giving the details. "Yeah, it's really cool. You get this tour guide. It costs like sixty dollars per person, and you get to drink beer and eat barbeque chicken when you're done."

I am thrilled and clap my hands together like a wound up little four-year-old.

"Let's do it, Heywood. I'm in!"

He then says it will be the Saturday of Memorial Day and he will be buying the tickets in advance so I should get the money to him soon. I look at the clock and realize I have to go teach my next pre-K class, but point at him as I leave and say, "Heywood, I'm in!"

He gives me the thumbs up and I excitedly realize I just sealed the deal.

～ ～ ～

May 2010—Memorial Day Weekend

We have Friday off from school, so I start to prepare what I am going to wear for the whitewater rafting trip. I know we will have to leave by

5:30 a.m. to get to Heywood's house by 6:30 a.m. From his house, it will take almost three hours to get to the Black River starting point. I begin trying on my bathing suits. I have five, so I figure one might work. I haven't had a bathing suit on since before my surgeries. This is the real thing. Dr. Panilio had promised he would make me look good in a bathing suit. I try on my black bikini. Oh my! I can see the scars underneath my arms and the halter top doesn't feel very supportive of "the girls."

The bottoms are worse. I've always worn high cut bikini bottoms to accentuate my long legs, but now they don't look good. My eyes are drawn to the scars in my groin area. The skin graft on my left leg, the one that had gotten infected, is extremely noticeable. It is quite the reddish brown color, and although the scar on the right leg is a thin line, it is still accentuated by the high-cut bikini bottoms. I try on the remainder of the bathing suits and then throw them on the floor. I sit naked on the bed and look in the mirror and begin to cry. Richard comes in and sits next to me.

"Aww honey, what's wrong?"

I toss my hand towards the little bikinis on the floor.

"Nothing looks good. Dr. Panilio lied; all you can see are my scars in those bathing suits."

Richard bends down and kisses the scar on my groin, then kisses the one on the right side of my chest. He sits up and kisses my lips and says, "You're beautiful."

I smile and wipe away my tears. Then Richard motions with his hand.

"Go buy a new bathing suit. It'll be good for you."

I agree that it will be healthy to buy a bathing suit that I feel and look good in. So I get dressed and head to an outdoor apparel outlet store which is only fifteen minutes from my home.

When I arrive, I immediately head over to the bathing suit section. I avoid every high-cut bikini and opt for the boy shorts and cute tankinis. I take two bathing suits into the dressing room: a black one with an adorable little empire waist belt; and a brown bathing suit that is babydoll style. I get naked and look at myself in the mirror and notice the scars don't look too bad when I don't have any clothes on. They appear worse when I wear clothes that draw attention to them.

I try on the black bathing suit first. Oh my! It looks beautiful, and more importantly, I feel beautiful in it. I think, *I'm definitely getting this one.* However, I went to the trouble of picking out the brown babydoll suit, so I figure I should at least try it on. So I do, and I love it too. One bathing suit I feel beautiful and wholesome in; the other I feel sexy in. I call Patty to tell her about my dilemma. I know what she'll tell me, but I think I better run it by someone, especially given the expensive price tags. She shouts in the phone at me: "Get both of them. It's priceless to feel that way."

Done! I make the decision to get both. I make the decision to feel beautiful and sexy again. I walk past the water shoes and one pair makes me turn my head. So I try them on. I feel athletic in them. They are blue Velcro, and not only are they water shoes, but you can walk in them comfortably as well. The black ones are contemporary and sporty. I text Patty with this next dilemma, and she immediately responds with, "You're worth it!"

When I get home, I try to sneak in with the big bag of new bathing suits and shoes, but Richard greets me on the porch with a cup of coffee in his hand. I smile and look down playfully, like I should be ashamed of myself for my shopping binge. He kisses my forehead and laughs as he adds, "This was way cheaper than psychotherapy."

I smile and ask him if he wants me to put on a fashion show for him. He rubs my bottom and whispers, "I'd love you to. Let's make sure the kids go to bed early."

I remind him that Adele is going to be staying over at Jennifer's house for the night and Matt is working. He sips his coffee, and, raising his eyebrow, says, "Even better."

～ ～ ～

The time comes around very quickly, and we are all ready for our big whitewater adventure. My friend Cheryl is at our house at 5:30, sharp. We all joke about how no one should be up this early, ever. I am happy my oldest friend is coming along, and she will be meeting my friends from school. She shows me the water suit she is going to wear for our big quest. I show her my new bathing suit, and then say our fashion show has to end here because we have to be at Heywood's house in Elmira by 6:30.

When we get to Heywood's house, we knock on the door, but there is no answer. I knock louder and yell, "Heywood, you up?"

Richard and I look at each other, and Cheryl asks, "I wonder if they left already."

I point to Heywood's vehicle in the driveway and say the other one is Val's car.

"They have to be here." I pound louder. "Val? Heywood? You guys up?" Then I cup my hands and yell up to the second floor. "Heywood!?"

At this point, we can hear people stomping around. Heywood opens up the door and rubs his eyes.

"Morning!"

Richard and I walk in, and I tease him.

"Heywood, rough night? This is so awesome! You overslept! Want me to make coffee?"

I then introduce him to Cheryl and continue to tease him endlessly, until Heywood's dad, Jeff, shows up. While Heywood and Val get ready, I ask Jeff how old he is. He informs all of us that he is seventy-five. I nudge my sixty-five-year-old husband and joke, "See, you're not the oldest one whitewater rafting!"

We take the Heywoods' minivan, which sits us all comfortably. Cheryl sits in the very back with Jeff. Richard and I sit in the mid-section. Heywood drives, and his wife Val sits up front with him. I am so happy Jeff and Cheryl are laughing and talking. Sometimes I get a little nervous, not knowing how people will connect, and a three-hour drive can feel more like an eight-hour trip. Today the conversations are warm and inviting, and our drive to Watertown is beautiful.

We arrive as many of my other colleagues are pulling into the side parking lot of the Black River touring company. The building is an old wooden warehouse, with yellow rafts piled on one side of the large open area. Vests and helmets are also piled near the rafts. We all gather in the parking lot in a circle, where I introduce Cheryl, Heywood introduces his dad, and some of the others introduce their spouses.

Heywood heads up to the ticket entrance and informs them that our teacher group is here. I notice some other groups appear by bus, and they all get off carrying water suits, looking like they know what they are doing. The only one with a water suit in our group is Cheryl, and I jokingly tell everyone that since this is Cheryl's third time whitewater rafting she will be on our raft.

Pam holds her stomach and whispers over to me, "I'm scared."

"This is going to be an awesome adventure. Don't worry! Be brave!" I hold my chest when I say it, adjusting "the girls" in their new black bathing suit and whispering, "Do you like my new bathing suit?"

She tells me she noticed it right away and asks how I am feeling. I roll my shoulders back and forth and say, "I'm excited to try this. You only live once!"

I have just realized that being brave has become my new motto with my new body and self. Actually, whitewater rafting is all new to me, and a few years ago no one would have ever used the words "whitewater rafting" and "Angela" in the same sentence. But this new me wants to try everything, even if it is just once.

All the groups are gathered in the parking lot and circle around. There is no mistaking which group is which, because each group has formed their own circle. A worker from the touring company comes out on the deck. He has dark sunglasses on and curly, crazy hair. He kind of looks like the groovy Greg Brady from *The Brady Bunch*, however this cool cat has a water suit on, and if I was a betting kind of gal, I'd bet he just burned a pin joint this morning. He has tattoos up and down his arm and he raises one arm up high and yells, "I need everyone to come to the back of the building for your quick class on whitewater rafting. Get geared up."

I am so excited. All the groups flock together and head to the back of the building. There is a large yellow raft centered on two pic-nic tables. The touring guide jumps up on it. This is his platform, and as he speaks I picture him doing this type of work as a reincarnated soul from the renaissance period. He is a natural Black River whitewa-ter rafting tour guide, a Hollywood personality who probably lives in his parent's basement.

"I'm Eric," he shouts out to the group, "and I'm one of your ten tour guides today." He points to the other nine characters standing next to the picnic tables, eight men and one tough woman, who also have dark sunglasses on, and then continues his rap. "You are in for a great adventure today. None of you will ever be the same again."

Everyone laughs at his spiel and I feel comfortable with the smiles coming from the other tour guides. Then Eric begins to talk about rules. This is where I, super responsible Angela, truly listen up.

"All joking aside, please let your tour guide know if there are any health issues or if you shouldn't whitewater raft today." He continues, "Seriously, folks, we have never lost anyone on our adventures. We have a comfortable waiting area and there are lots of things to do around Watertown. So, if you are not physically fit to help your group—because this is a real group effort—you need to let your tour guide know."

On and on he goes. I bend to my right and whisper to Richard, who is standing next to me.

"Do you think it's okay that I go?"

Richard nods. "You're fine."

Then I bend to my left and whisper to Heywood.

"Heywood, I'm not going to be very helpful. I'm still quite sore, but I really want to go."

"You're good, don't say anything," he whispers back.

After Eric makes everyone laugh and provides all the rules and regulations in a serious manner, or as serious as a stoned whitewater rafting tour guide can, he tells the groups to gather with their guides.

Richard and I agree that we, along with Cheryl, should go with the Heywood family, for a total of seven in our raft—six of us and our tour guide. Our tour guide has long blonde hair and a long blonde mustache that twirls off to the sides. He has a Yosemite Sam "shoot 'em down" type of air about him. He is a medium-statured, tough-looking guy, and he flicks his cigarette to the ground. Stepping on it he says, "Okay, gang, you're with me. My name is Rocky." Then he motions us to our raft.

He checks our helmets and vests and then gives mine a little tug to tighten it up. "You need this good and snug, sweetie."

I close my eyes and smile because I don't want him to see the slight pain he has just inflicted on my chest. I can't wait to be on our way because once we are, I know I will be good to go on. I won't have to wait for my friends in some comfortable area.

Rocky sits at the front of the raft and gives instructions on how we will use our paddles for moving away from rocks and things that could hurt us. He stresses the importance of everyone using all they have to help the group paddle safely. It feels like forever before we actually get to glide off into the Black River. I look over at the other tour guides giving their instructions with their crews. I notice there are four separate men in kayaks. They will be travelling along with all of us. They are the safety crew and they are already doing stunts with their kayaks and laughing with one another. In a weird sort of way I feel completely safe with this crazy crew. I can tell this is the job they do day in and day out. Yes, maybe they're high, but they know what they are doing.

Before I know it, we are off and floating down the Black River. I raise my paddle and yell to my friends in the raft behind us. "We're going down the Black River!"

They whoop it up and raise their paddles too, and even the groups that we don't know raise their paddles and yell back to us as well. I feel like part of a big clan. This experience is already making my new self stronger.

At first it is just mostly padoodling down the river, listening to our tour guide, Rocky, rant about how he grew up on this river and has trained every tour guide here. He knows this river inside and out, like the back of his hand. He's been doing this job for over twenty-eight years, he says, and his girlfriend is the one and only "lady" that works as a tour guide for this company. On and on Rocky talks, and I listen to it mostly out of politeness. I feel snug with my husband, the Heywoods, and Cheryl, who's sitting directly behind me.

I mostly notice the birds flying up above in the beautiful bright blue sky. I take in a gorgeous blue heron that flies low enough to make me wonder about pterodactyls during the dinosaur era. That's how large and beautiful they seem to me. The water sparkles with sun diamonds everywhere and I inhale deeply as I take in the moment.

Soon the river begins to get much narrower. I then start to carefully listen to Rocky as he mentions the Black River gorge. He speaks up over the now loud water rapids, "You are going to need those paddles for this upcoming ledge and boulder. As a reminder, a lot of this will be Class IV rapids. There's no sitting back. The real work will be in the set of Hole Brothers, and Knife's Edge." He laughs adding, "Wait until we get to the Zig-Zag and then the Cruncher. Whoa! I still find it exciting."

I say to our group, giving them quite the anxiety-ridden laugh, "Okay, this is pretty bad when our tour guide, who has been doing this for twenty-eight years, still finds it exciting."

"Little lady, I love this place," says Rocky. "It's always changing." He points to the cliff with a newly fallen tree. "You have to watch out for new things happening all the time."

I think about the profoundness of his last statement. I close my eyes and feel the warm sunshine on my face.

"Use your oars, move away from that boulder," Rocky yells.

I put my oar in the water, trying to do what he is telling us to do, but my chest still hurts. Between the other five people working hard, and knowing what I'd been through with all my operations, I don't feel bad for not using all of my strength. At least not until we get to Knife's Edge, where Rocky looks right back at me. In front of everyone, he points at me and says, "Little lady, you need to help. Use that oar, paddle and push with it. This is a team effort." He turns away and everyone gets really quiet.

Heywood looks back at me and shakes his head no to me and whispers, "Don't worry about it."

I am worried though. I want to do what I can. If I told Rocky beforehand about my four operations, I was afraid he wouldn't let me go. Therefore, I try to push and paddle more on the trip.

When we are about half way through our trip, we come to a shale plateau. All of the groups tie off their rafts to a fallen tree. Everyone gets out of their rafts and mingles. I love seeing everyone laugh and smile and connect. There is a metal cooler on the center of the large shale island. One of the tour guides begins to pass out a snack which is wrapped in foil. My husband grabs one for me. They are peanut butter tortilla wraps with oat cereal and honey. I take mine over by our tour guide who is eating alone on a big boulder.

"Hey!" I say looking at him to see if he will welcome me.

"Hey," he replies while chewing his food. I look around to see if anyone will hear what I am going to say.

"Rocky, I need to tell you something. I recently had a mastectomy and three other operations. I don't mean not to pull my weight on this trip, but I still get sore when I make certain movements."

Rocky's face morphs from grim Yosemite Sam to a compassionate, gentle soul.

"Oh my God! Why didn't you tell me?"

I start to tear up. "I was afraid you wouldn't let me come along."

He touches my arm. "My mom died from breast cancer."

I start to explain how I don't have cancer and I can tell that my genetic disposition is too much for Rocky to understand. He misunderstands me and thinks I *used* to have cancer. I see the confusion, so I try another quick *BRCA1* lesson, but he still thinks I used to have cancer. Once I realize he isn't comprehending my fast *BRCA1* tutorial, I just stop and smile at him. I know he understands cancer. I let Rocky believe what he is going to believe. He transforms into a caring, thoughtful human being the remainder of the trip. Rocky goes a little overboard on the kindness towards me, but I graciously take that in as well.

After doing the set of Hole Brothers and Zig-Zag, we come up on the crazy Cruncher. Rocky explains how water will most likely get up everyone's noses. He then winks, points to a big slate boulder, and whispers over to me, "You can hang on this rock while your group does this if you want."

So I do. I get out of the boat and watch my crew paddle against the current and into a whitewater ravine. While watching their madness, I look up at the gorge ahead of them and see an osprey fly over with a fish in its mouth. I begin to cry and laugh, almost uncontrollably. I can't believe that I have just whitewater rafted down the Black River. I can't believe all that I have done to date: the mastectomy, the hysterectomy, the reconstruction process, and now the whitewater rafting trip. This adventure on this warm spring day, surrounded by the love of my closest friends, and yes, even Rocky's newfound compassion, makes my heart open ten times greater that very moment.

I am watching Richard in the raft with my friends. I feel safe in Rocky's hands. All of it makes me feel alive and present in openness. I am grateful for the water rapids being so loud because no one can hear me crying my loud tears of joy. If anything, they can only see me laughing with my beaming smile, ear to ear. My teary eyes are hidden behind my dark sunglasses. And at this point, it doesn't matter if anyone sees. However, Rocky notices my tears, and comes over to me.

"Are you okay there, lady?" he asks.

I wipe my tears and laugh. "Tears of joy!"

He touches my arm, then looks at our crew and crosses his arms in front of his chest. He nods a masculine nod to keep back any tears he has.

The groups finish their last whitewater section and we continue down the Black River. It widens and mini waterfalls can be seen off in the distant gorges. Everything is beautiful. All of our group's rafts are now hooked together onto one powerboat, which has a cooler of drinks for everyone.

Richard grabs a soda and I grab a beer. I can sense everyone's exhaustion during the calm and now quiet ride back to the warehouse.

I yell up to the sun.

"Nostrovia."

People laugh and some hold their drinks up and echo my call up into the beautiful gorge.

"Nostrovia!"

"What does 'nostrovia' mean?" Rocky asks.

"It's Polish. It means 'to your health'!"

He holds up his beer to me, "To your health, little lady. Nostrovia!"
We smile at each other and I snuggle into my husband.

We get back to the warehouse where a chicken barbeque awaits us, with lots of potato salad, beans, and beer. Cheryl is walking around the tented tables, asking my teacher friends, "When are we going to do this again?"

I can hear some respond "Never again" and "Once is enough."

I head into the gift store and buy a pink T-shirt that reads, "I paddle, I sing, I live!" A perfect ending to a perfect day!

～～～

December 2010
My friend Jennifer and I always have our semi-annual luncheon. Her birthday is in December and mine is in June. In lieu of buying needless gifts for one another, we opt to buy lunch for one another. This tradition of ours has been going on for years. We both realize that time is more precious than any gift. Our lunch usually involves lots of red wine, a dessert, oh and yes, a lunch in between. Did I mention wine? Also our meal is usually three or more hours followed by needless excessive shopping. It has become a tradition I can't seem to live without. Jennifer and I connect so deeply. We are like sisters. She is super responsible like me. She can juggle multiple priorities and projects at once. That is why I chose her to take care of my daughter during my operations.

Jennifer has a degree in travel and tourism, and is a co-owner of an aviation company, so she knows how to plan a vacation. During our luncheon, and after our second glass of wine, she asks, "Well, now that you're like bionic woman, what do you say we take our baby girls on a little vacation?"

"What do you have in mind?"

She pulls out her smart phone and we figure our calendars mesh together well with February's school break. We talk about the indoor water park that is only about three hours from where we live. It is in Erie, Pennsylvania. I tell Jennifer how Adele has wanted to go to this water park. I laugh as I explain how Adele told me this, way back on that very first day I came home from my mastectomy. I laugh harder remembering that moment, and how far I have come since that day. I explain how Adele had excitedly said, "I think we should go to Splash Lagoon!"

Jennifer sips her wine. "Let's do it!"

I know Jennifer will put it all together. I will just have to pack our things and bring a bottle of wine for our nightly hotel room talk. Then we clink our wine glasses together and drink more.

Over Christmas break I tell Adele that I have one more gift for her. "What is it?" she asks excitedly.

I bring her to my computer and let her sit on my lap while I pull up Splash Lagoon's website, which includes a short video. I press play and we watch it together. Afterwards I hug her and say, "Guess what? Remember way back. Last December, when I got out of the hospital, you said maybe when I was feeling better, that we could go to Splash Lagoon. Well, we're going!"

Her eyes get big and she eagerly claps her hands together. "When?"

I tell her over February break. She seems disappointed that it isn't right now. I rub her back and explain that it will be here before she knows it.

Then we look at all the slides and attractions. Adele points to the biggest waterslide.

"I want to go down that one, Hurricane Hole. Will you go down it with me?"

It looks completely scary, and that is from sitting behind a computer looking at it on a small screen. I hug her and pretend I am frightened.

"We'll see."

Sure enough, February break is here in no time and we are on our way to Splash Lagoon. I pile my bags in the back of Jennifer's car, and her daughter Sabrina and Adele sit in the back. Both of them have their headphones on and I tell them that, since it is a long drive, perhaps we can limit our electronic devices. This trip is about "girl power," and I hold my arms up in my victory stance. They laugh, and I wink at Jennifer. Our trip there is delightful. Jen and I talk and talk; about our husbands, about our parents, about our children, about everything under the sun. The three hour trip is virtually effortless.

When we get to Splash Lagoon, the girls' eyes are big. We all carry our over abundant luggage for our one night and two day stay and joke that if we were staying any longer we would have had to rent a semitruck. We check in and look at our hotel room first. We are staying at one of the adjoining hotels that is attached to the entrance of Splash Lagoon. The hotel room is absolutely adorable. It has a set of bunk beds with a separating wall up the side, which gives the illusion of the girls having their own room. They have a countertop with a television set and the separating wall has pictures of fish under the ocean.

Jen and I pile our things on our side of the room, which has a queen-sized bed and a large television set on a desk. We all quickly decide to get our bathing suits on, pack some snacks, and head down to Splash Lagoon. As we come upon the entrance, I can smell the chlorine. When Jennifer opens the door, we can hardly believe our eyes. The water park is larger than we had imagined. There are tons of people going every which way in the eighty degree, glassed-in park. They are all laughing and screaming and it all echoes playfully in the three story palm tree décor.

Jen and I look at each other as if to say, "Now what?" Then I point towards some tables.

"Let's stick together and find a table to base at, just in case one of us gets lost. We can always return back to the table."

We carry our towels and snack bag and find a perfect table under a palm tree umbrella. Sabrina points to the biggest and baddest waterslide, Hurricane Hole, and yells "Come on mom, let's go on that one!"

We laugh and explain to the girls that we should work our way up to going down that one. We then head over to a double tube slide, one in which we can go down with our girls together. Later, we individually get floats and hang at the Lazy River, where I can view every waterslide in the park. As I float, I notice how everyone who just finished coming down a waterslide has a smile. I also notice how everyone who comes off the biggest slide, Hurricane Hole, is bursting with laughter. I think, *I have been through so much serious stuff this past year, I need to have fun.*

I yell over to Jen, who is floating just ahead of me on the Lazy River. "Hey, let's take the girls down Hurricane Hole!"

She laughs. "Really?"

She looks up to the three-story stairs and notices the line is shorter than all the other slides. "Okay," she shouts back. She then yells to the girls, who are on a double tube in front of her. "Bri, let's go down Hurricane Hole."

Adele looks scared, and at first she doesn't want to go down it. I reassure her. I tell her we will go first and if she doesn't want to go down it, she can walk back down the stairs. All she has to do is tell the lifeguard that she is scared and doesn't want to do it.

I can tell that the only reason why she agrees to go is because she has a way out. We all get out of the Lazy River and put our inner tubes up. I rub my hands together and excitedly cheer, "Let's do this!"

Deep inside, I feel so awesome showing my daughter how to be brave. Going down Hurricane Hole is symbolic. It is not just about being brave enough to do a water park ride. Rather, it is my message to her that you must be brave in this world when you make a decision. Be brave and don't waver back and forth and hem and haw. Be brave and do it. Or, as my cousin Jim had said to me well over a year ago, just before my mastectomy, "A mediocre decision in a timely manner is better than a perfect decision made too late."

When we get to the top of the slide, I jokingly push Jen's shoulder. "You go first."

She laughs and then looks at her daughter. "Bri, I'll wait for you at the bottom."

Before she gets onto the slide, I point to the diagram and remind her how we should position ourselves as we go down the slide. The picture shows a stick figure with arms crossed over its chest. Of course this is quite appropriate for me.

Jen goes first, and we can all hear her scream even when she is halfway through. All of our eyes meet as we listen to her. Sabrina goes next and doesn't scream at all.

When it is my turn, I look at Adele and say, "Be brave!" I cross my arms over my newly reconstructed chest and go down Hurricane Hole.

Now, let me explain why this is called Hurricane Hole. First, you wind around and around, and this winding happens quickly in a dark tunnel, where you can't see a thing and only hear the echoes of your own screaming and laughing. Then, when you have come out of the dark tunnel, you are in an open vortex. This is where you start to slow down from the ride. However, once you are in the vortex, you realize you are swirling slowly towards the center of the vortex, where there is no bottom. So you become progressively terrified during this part of the ride. You will undoubtedly fall out the bottom and into a deep pool where you have to swim to a young teenage lifeguard that will hopefully help you out if you need it. Crazy!

When my body comes out into the open vortex, my arms don't stay crossed over my chest like in the diagram we just looked at. I instinctively sit up, laughing in a panic, and then my bathing suit bottom catches on something in the hard plastic. Or does it catch on the ring on my finger? I don't know, but I am flapping around like a fish out of water, so I am not sure what the heck I've caught it on. Regardless, it rips a hole in the rear of my suit. I am joyously scared as I fall through the hole into a deep pool. I come up to the surface coughing and laughing with water up my nose.

Jennifer and Bri are laughing and ready to aid the lifeguard to help me out. "I'm okay!" I say.

Then I quickly remember Adele is up there. I stand there with Jennifer and Bri and momentarily wonder if the next person will be my daughter, or if she chose to walk back down the three story flight of stairs. We wait and wait. I hold my breath. Then, *splash*, through the hole comes Adele. We all clap our hands and cheer for Adele. She swims to the side laughing and coughing too. When she comes out of the deep pool, we all high five each other and I hug Adele and whisper in her ear, "You're so brave! Good decision, don't ya think?!"

Her lips are slightly purple and her eyebrows are water drenched. My heart melts when she looks at me with her big brown eyes. She smiles and nods her head excitedly. "Uh-huh!" Then she fearlessly adds, "Let's do it again!"

"Let's do it!" I cheer our bravery onward.

This day we go back down Hurricane Hole three more times.

~ ~ ~

I love who I have become. I have honed in on my spontaneity. My spirit has been strengthened by understanding who I am genetically and who I want to now be emotionally. This is the one reason why I can be grateful for being *BRCA1* positive. Before I found out I was *BRCA1* positive, I was going through life on autopilot. I had moments of true meaning, however my days were not spent feeling the true value of life and how all things are connected in this big universe of ours.

Being *BRCA1* positive has helped me bravely salute anything I have to tackle, and do so head on. Once my surgeries are complete, this is when my life adventures really start. I write myself my own prescription, "to live fully." My year of healing and recovery includes so much more, everything from whitewater rafting, Splash Lagoon's Hurricane Hole, roller coasters with 208 foot drops, and presenting my first two educational books to teachers across the country. Driving to Nashville with my oldest friend, Cheryl, so I can present both of my educational books to one of the largest NAFCC conferences in the country . . . well that's another bold story altogether.

All of these adventures have shaped me into a new woman that excitedly shouts, "I want to try everything in this life at least once." My behavior over the next year is like an ongoing recovery party. I am ready to do other adventurous things; not just once, but three or four times.

Here's to living life regardless of whatever your genetic disposition holds. Here's to celebrating and finding meaning and purpose in even the smallest things. Here's to all the decisions we make. Here's to the personal decisions we make to live our best life. NOSTROVIA!

Epilogue

I made these very personal decisions—to have genetic testing, then a preventative mastectomy and a hysterectomy—because of where I was in my forty-one-year-old life. First, my age was a critical factor in making these imperative decisions. As everyone is now keenly aware, cancer and early death are a vile part of my family. My dad had died at forty-two, and his mother at forty-seven; my mom had died at fifty-two, and her mother at fifty-two as well. My uncle John died young too. Therefore, age was fundamental in considering all my pressing decisions.

Next, I thought I was finished with having children. This was an important issue when thinking of preventative operations; I already had two beautiful children, Adele and Matthew. Shortly after my hysterectomy, there was another surprise: my husband and I made the decision to adopt. Okay, this wasn't just a surprise, it was a BIG SURPRISE! In a nutshell, a baby was born to my sister, and since my sister still struggled with taking care of herself, her little baby girl needed a family and a home. The moment I felt sad that I couldn't have any more children, this was the instant the universe again gave me exactly what I needed. We got Holly when she was only one month old. By the time *Angela's Decision* is first available to you, Holly will be three, Adele fourteen, and Matthew will be twenty-four years old. It was not only ironic how my family got bigger after my hysterectomy decision, but very touching as well.

Then of course there were also all the other decisions in between. What type of surgery to have, what medication choices, the reconstruction options, and all the alternative healing preferences, all of which were extremely delicate and personal issues. The important part here is to note that these are personal decisions. Clearly, when confronted with any critical decision you need to make, they will be your very own, made in line with what is perfectly right for you and your life. Genetic testing, preventative surgeries, high surveillance health screenings, or even to do nothing, is a decision—are all decisions—you might make. These decisions are yours and yours alone. Remember, no one has to walk in your shoes but you.

Blessings to you on every decision you make!

Wholeheartedly,

Angela Schmidt Fishbaugh

Resources

- **American Cancer Society**
  http://www.cancer.org/
  (800) 227-2345

- **Breastcancer.org**
  http://www.breastcancer.org/
  (610) 642-6550

- **Bright Pink**
  http://www.brightpink.org/

- **FORCE: Facing Our Risk of Cancer Empowered**
  http:// www.facingourrisk.org/
  (866) 288-RISK (7475)

  For clinical trials and research opportunities:
  http://www.facingourrisk.org/information_research/overview.php

- **Living Beyond Breast Cancer**
  http://www.lbbc.org/
  (855) 807-6386
  mail@lbbc.org

- **National Cancer Institute at the National Institutes of Health**
  http://www.cancer.gov/
  (800) 4-CANCER (226237)

- **Sharsheret**
  http://www.sharsheret.org/
  (866) 474-2774
  info@sharsheret.org

- **The University of Pennsylvania's Basser Research Center for BRCA**
  http://www.penncancer.org/basser/
  (215) 662-2748
  basserinfo@uphs.upenn.edu

Acknowledgments

First, I would like to give special recognition to my Skyhorse Publishing editor, Andres Dietz-Chavez, for helping me to shine. I will be forever grateful for your hard work and extra efforts! I'd like to also thank Constance Renfrow for our initial connection. A special thank you to all those at Skyhorse Publishing who joined in making this book a helpful resource for all women.

I am also blessed to have so many wonderful friends, family, and colleagues on my journey. Your combined love and support throughout my decision making process made my recovery a blessed one. My old-time friends, namely Jennifer, Cheryl, and Maureen, all of whom I've known for virtually my whole life, are my beloved confidants and angels from heaven.

I need to also thank my family for their long distance love: my Aunt Eva, Aunt Deb, and my cousin Jim, who always knows how to make me laugh on any given day. I am forever thankful to my brother Ben for being my best friend growing up. I will eternally love my sister for giving me the greatest gift she could ever give. Love to my brother, Anthony, the one who continually reminds all of us of our past. We always can count on you to recall the exact day and time that anything ever happened. Thank you to all my family for your sustenance.

I need to acknowledge my godmother, for our tri-weekly phone conversations about cooking, cleaning, gardening, Bob, my kids, my husband, the pets, the next get together, the next shopping trip, sewing, our projects, nothing, something, everything, the holidays, and mostly for keeping our Polish heritage alive. I couldn't ask for a more devoted godmother. I am further grateful for my beautiful children, Holly, Adele, and Matthew (or "HAM"), for all of the delightful Chutzpah that you offer this world. God I love you!

My besties from work: Heywood, Pam, and Patty; and all my colleagues who celebrate with me—I wouldn't be the same without you. Whether we are celebrating at our annual "pitch your tent night," under our big sky, at a family party, or a book festivity, thank you for being there for me. Also, I cannot thank enough each and every staff member who prepared meals for my family so we didn't have to cook for a whole month during my recovery. Your sunshine is "highly effective." I love you, my friends.

I am very grateful for everyone mentioned in this book. The great moments, the not so good times; all of it strengthened me in some way. I want to give special recognition to all my healthcare professionals, who helped me with their expertise, sensitivity, and openness; and, for Terry who offered me her Qigong services so I could nourish my body back to balance.

I could never acknowledge my husband enough. Richard, I am exceptionally blessed to be on this journey with you. I cherish your truth, respect your path, and love you with all my heart and soul. Thank you for being such a good, good man. Thank you for helping our children as they make their best decisions in this world. I am a better person because of you.

Thank you, Nostrovia, and Namaste!